# BRIGIE

*'It's the only thing that kills girls her age. Boys kill themselves on motorbikes and girls die of this'*

A harsh way to tell a mother that her beautiful, gregarious, fun-loving sixteen-year-old daughter has an incurable and agonising form of cancer. That she has three months to live . . .

But Janet Taylor is no ordinary person, nor was her daughter Brigie. Both wanted to know the truth, as early as possible. Brigie confronted this dreadful knowledge with laughter, dignity and unfailing courage, sustained not only by her fighting spirit but by an inner peace. Her mother's honest account of Brigie's calm composure in the face of death, and of her bravery in suffering, is a poignant tribute to a remarkable girl.

'A wise, inspiring and heart-warming story that will surely strengthen and comfort others'.

*Sunday Express*

'No one could fail to be gripped and inspired, and perhaps radically changed too, by this honestly written, heartfelt book'.

*Good Housekeeping*

*About the Author*

Janet Taylor was born and grew up in New Zealand. She taught English in secondary schools there, and in England, after coming here in 1956. She now runs a small post office in the Yorkshire Dales.

# Brigie
# A Life: 1965–1981

# Janet Taylor

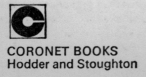

CORONET BOOKS
Hodder and Stoughton

*The author and publishers wish to thank
Faber and Faber Ltd. for permission to quote
from 'East Coker' from* Four Quartets *by T. S.
Eliot and to David Higham Associates Ltd. for
permission to quote from 'And death shall
have no dominion' by Dylan Thomas, in*
Collected Poems, *published by J. M. Dent.*

First published in 1984 by
Hodder & Stoughton Ltd.

Coronet edition 1985.

**British Library C.I.P.**

Taylor, Janet, *1931–*
    Brigie: a life: 1965–1981.——(Coronet books)
    1. Cancer——Psychological aspects
    2. Terminally ill——Psychology
    I. Title
    362.1'96994        RC262

ISBN 0 340 37180 3

Printed and bound in Great Britain for
Hodder and Stoughton Paperbacks, a
division of Hodder and Stoughton Ltd.,
Mill Road, Dunton Green, Sevenoaks,
Kent (Editorial Office: 47 Bedford
Square, London, WC1 3DP) by
Cox & Wyman Ltd., Reading

This book is dedicated to all those families who will face a similar experience. When they too feel the intense pain, may they know as well the wonder and the blessing.

# Notes

Brigie's full name was Brigid, but the pronunciation of her name in the family was 'Bridgie'. Her school friends in Skipton called her Brigie with a hard 'g'. The initials G.M. and G. are used to distinguish between her father, Geoffrey Moorhouse, and my husband and her stepfather, Geoffrey Taylor. Children's spellings in diary entries and letters are retained.

# Acknowledgments

I am grateful to the late Bishop John Robinson for permission to print his funeral address, and to family and friends who allowed me to use their letters and accounts of visits. I am grateful to all who have made helpful and encouraging comments and especially to Amanda Batten of Hodder and Stoughton for her thoughtful and sensitive editing. The advice and help given by my husband, Geoffrey, has been invaluable and is matched only by his involvement and good humour in the typing of a very untidy manuscript.

# Contents

# Introduction

When Brigie died in December 1981 I felt a very strong
compulsion to write down everything I could remember
about her illness and dying. Losing a child had always seemed
to me the worst disaster that could happen, and yet her
courage and calm acceptance of it, and our own new closeness
around her, turned it into an experience which was beautiful
and profound, and I wanted to make a record for the family
so that none of us would forget any detail of it. As I started
writing I realised that I was talking not just to them: there
was a compelling need to share this experience with a much
wider group, with all who fear death, especially for the
young. It soon became clear also that if the end had meaning,
so had the whole life from its beginning.

I have tried to write down everything that happened as I
saw it, or as related by others, and not to gloss over any of the
difficulties. The only omissions that I am aware of are a few
details of conversation which would be hurtful to individuals.
This is a very personal account, and I did not see everything,
nor can I judge what it was really like for others involved.
What was undoubtedly true was that a lively sixteen-year-
old girl, taken in the full flush of her teenage obsessions and
with no previously obvious spiritual resources, came to accept
death peacefully. As one religiously sceptical member of the
family said, 'She was certainly drawing on something.' I

believe that a power of love and goodness reached her and us and that we are all, in a very strange way, stronger for having experienced it.

Janet Taylor
February 1983

# 1

## Over-the-back and beyond

We spent Brigie's early years in Broxbourne, part of London's commuter belt, and ours was one in a row of early Victorian houses built by a City magnate for his executives when the railway line was first extended out from Liverpool Street. In those spacious days, I was told, when business was more leisurely and the journey faster, the City gentlemen would come home for lunch to their rural retreat, beyond the mill and the church by the river, and with an uninterrupted view to a few other handsome old houses among the surrounding fields, farms and woods. By the early 1960s all that had been changed by the urban sprawl of the thirties: no longer did a dairy herd cross the Cambridge road to be milked night and morning, and the old pub down the road in Hoddesdon, where Izaak Walton stayed on his fishing expeditions to the River Lea, was pulled down soon after we arrived to make way for a supermarket. Our first window cleaner could remember better times: 'This used to be quite a high-class area,' he said unguardedly, 'before people such as yourselves started moving in.' The Churchfields houses, even so, retained a certain dignity despite the disappearance of Victorian formalities: they had the moulded ceilings and the high skirting-boards, the service bells by the fireplace, the heavy panelled doors, and the ancient gas lamp-holders that gave a feeling of history and solidity. I sometimes thought, as the

13

tide of children and toys threatened to engulf us, of my unknown Victorian predecessor with her no doubt orderly ways and her servant in the kitchen, and wondered what she would have made of the chaos of building blocks and Matchbox cars all over her dining-room floor. For our more casual way of life, though, it was a house where children could grow up without feeling cramped or hemmed in.

This was just as well when all the neighbouring children poured through the door, as they did at least once a week by arrangement, and then the space seemed limited enough. We joined in the informal play-group system of the road, which meant that one mother, at least, was sometimes free to have a day off, or organise a children's party, or simply do the shopping. This semi-communal life had advantages for the children, too: there was always someone to play with, a different house to be in, new things to see. A close-knit little community became established and the sharing helped us all over many a minor crisis, and some major ones too.

Nor was children's play confined to houses and gardens, for at Churchfields we had 'over-the-back' as we called it, a wasteland behind the brick walls of our back gardens which years before had been quarried for gravel. When we lived there it was all humps and hollows, trees had grown again and there were masses of blackberries. For children it was magical: a small kingdom of fabulous places with names like 'the witches' tunnel' and 'the long grass'. There they endlessly built their 'camps' and lived their games of make-believe in secret hide-aways among the crowding bushes and the old man's beard. Here we had our neighbourhood bonfire every November 5th, when they would tear through the tracks in the undergrowth with their sparklers, loving to be afraid of the dark. The only limit to freedom there was that you couldn't go through the railings on the far side where the New River flowed, but that apart it was a glorious small safe world of liberty. It was a great day when the latest small child in the road was deemed old enough to go over-the-back to play, an intermediate step towards the real outside world, because here they had to learn to cope with occasional hostile forces like the bigger boys from round the corner (nicknamed the 'Skinnies') who invaded their territory and broke down their camps, or simply their older brothers and sisters who spied on them and giggled at their make-believe talk.

Brigie was born at home on a Sunday, January 17th, 1965, and within half an hour Jane and Andrew were in to see her in her cot. We wondered what they would make of this new sister, who quite early on showed that she could be vociferous and demanding in spite of her size. It was possible that Andrew might feel displaced in no longer being the youngest, and G.M. and Aunty Lucy, a favourite adopted aunt in joint charge of the household, were at pains to keep everything normal for them, and Linda, the midwife, was a success too, because she taught them to make soap bubbles when she bathed them. Andrew, in fact, was mildly interested in the baby, but mostly got on with the more serious business of playing with his friend, Tim. It was Jane, at four and a half, who came to feel that this new person, while delightful as a baby, was a threat to her as a sister. She found her own way of asserting herself in the weeks that followed: refusing to leave the house or to let me go out either, and it was a struggle, later on, to persuade her to allow Brigie's baptism to happen. This was to be in Derby where Canon Paul Miller, her prospective godfather, lived in the Bridge Chapel House. He suggested that he baptise her in the tiny chapel which opened out of his sitting room. Gladys and Dick, her grandparents, travelled over from Lancashire with their daughter, Lesley, and Lucy, who were her godmothers. It was a beautiful place for the short family service, during which Paul lit a baptismal candle and placed it on the altar. Afterwards he gave it, just half-burnt, to G.M. to keep, possibly to be relit at her confirmation, he suggested.

Jane gradually regained her confidence, but the pattern of behaviour was beginning to take shape. Andrew would seem to take life more calmly, 'a good solid citizen', someone called him, and Jane's imagination would open up possibilities of threat and havoc. She was a dreamy child, a bit like me in feeling large and clumsy among her contemporaries, and especially in relation to Brigie, who grew into a pretty little thing, knowing exactly what she wanted and how to get it. This seemingly supreme self-confidence and capacity to manage events set her slightly apart in the family. After Michael was born, fifteen months later, a round and amiable character, everyone's favourite (Jane did not feel threatened by *him*), Brigie was often the odd one out, her essentially female characteristics giving an abrasiveness and sharpness to our family life. Though small, she fought tenaciously for her 'rights', loud in her protests at the others' teasings and gibes.

Her distinct personality is remembered by others. A neighbour of that time wrote: 'I loved Brigie and have one particular and happy picture of her in your playroom at No. 18, her own very self-contained little person, being regal and proud of Michael's arrival.' Another friend wrote: 'I have one memory I keep turning to in particular, of a dainty little girl of, I think, three, explaining to me with the utmost gravity on some matter of responsible behaviour, I forget just what, "I'm a big girl. Michael's only little." '

The loosely communal life we lived there probably helped our children to cope with the break-up of their parents' marriage: it certainly helped me. We were careful to avoid creating any conflict of loyalties between us, and whatever private griefs there were, at least the outward life went on much as before. My father was still there, Pompah to the children, a reassuringly predictable figure in a world of change. He would be with them for hours, nursing an irritable baby, or walking the pushchair when they got bigger. For Brigie he had a special place; she was the first grandchild he had seen from the beginning, and she was a girl. His own strict Scottish upbringing made it hard for him to tolerate the freedom these children, particularly the boys, enjoyed, and as they all got bigger, girls as well as boys, and began to assert themselves or to interfere with his garden, relations were often strained. For all his crustiness, though, Pompah was a man of integrity, and the bond that he established with the children when they were small helped to temper the irritations of later years. He lived with us for seventeen years, until a fortnight before his death in 1978, and they look back on him now, I think, with a mixture of affection and amusement at his funny ways; a powerful personality, looking like the old New Zealand sheep farmer that he still felt himself to be, and proud of his grandchildren, even though he often disapproved of their behaviour.

In her early years particularly Brigie had a strong bond with him. This helped, I think, to develop a softer side to her personality which might otherwise have lain dormant. At times when impotent fury and frustration would consume her small person, he would succeed in distracting her. 'Come on, Brig,' he would say, 'we'll just sit here and look at the book. Come on now, you can do it. *You* know all about it.' And the angry, fairy-like creature would hold his horny finger as it travelled across the page and peace would return. As she got older and more assertive, even with him, the bond loosened, and she was often impatient with him, but near her own death she thought she saw Pompah sitting in the chair. Was he there to help and reassure her?

When I try now to hold a mental picture of the three-year-old Brigie, I see most clearly the slightly curly, wispy hair and the delicately defined features set either in fierce determination or gleeful triumph. The nose had already learnt to sniff in derision. Our battles about shoes must have started very early as I remember her at two and a half insisting on wearing over-large flip-flops that came off every two steps. One could not help laughing at this tenacious small person, and the dignity with which she would assert her position. She was very affronted with me after some argument when she was about three, and announced that she was 'leaving home', appearing later carrying a cumbersome load of treasures, including her small cane chair. When I asked her why she was taking that, she gave me a withering look. 'To sit on,' she said with high scorn, and set her mouth grimly with the triple effort of carrying her bundle, keeping her flip-flops on, and retaining her dignity. Jane met her down the road that day, and brought her back very solicitously, telling me that I had been very nasty and unkind to Brigie, and made a great fuss of her for the next ten minutes. Brigie basked in the attention from this unexpected quarter and treated me with disdain. She could triumph over her friends as well, coming along the path from school one day holding hands in an uncharacteristically demonstrative show of affection for her friend's best friend, indicating with her small smile of triumph that we should all realise who was in charge.

Her friends would look on in awe at these decisive acts, and many of them were wary of her. As Andrew commented later, 'She had a tongue like a knife.' School days were a carefree time, punctuated with the small events of childhood. When it came to sports days Brigie had no great incentive to win; while her brothers became quite athletic and good at games, and Jane could be persuaded to play for her side, Brigie, disliking strenuous physical effort, was proof against moral appeals to help her 'house' or play for the school. She went to the swimming club every week with the others, and learned to swim strongly, but resented the number of lengths they were expected to accomplish. Birthday parties were much more to her taste, especially her own; she got all the presents.

Brigie had no great difficulty with school work and went through none of the traumas with sums that Jane experienced. On the other hand there was no great academic success either, and her main accomplishments were achieved with little effort. That was how she liked it. Her favourite teacher, Miss Grafham, was very enthusiastic once about her singing. She had never heard a small child keep so unerringly in tune, she said, and Brigie found the recorder easy and therefore enjoyable. Her judgments on the teachers who did not measure up to Miss Grafham's special qualities were harsh and unqualified. 'She's a cow,' was an epithet which started then and was still being applied in other places, long after she left junior school.

She always appeared to have a great deal of self-confidence and capacity to dominate in a small group, but she never aspired to leadership in a wider sense. Her self-possession could be unnerving to some of her more uncertain contemporaries, but she would always assert in later years that she was really quite shy. If that was the case she managed to cover it up very effectively.

She must have felt shy when G. first came to Churchfields, but from the kitchen I could hear her giving him a long and piping exposition about something, in contrast to the silent Michael. He taught her to play chess and was impressed by her sharpness and quick percipience, not just in the matter of games. That sharpness, however, was not always an easy quality to live with. It became more evident as G. and I began spending more time together: her violin became the first weapon in her armoury. She and Ellen and Emma had started lessons a year before when they were about seven. The drive, of course, came from their mothers, and with such small children it was necessary to be with them during their lessons and their practice, spending a lot of time encouraging the small bows to find the right notes. Her teacher found her progress very promising. She accepted the praise with seeming indifference. She was learning the violin simply because I wanted her to, and though pleased by her merit pass in Grade II when she was nine, she never developed a love of the instrument which would carry her over into working on her own. As long as I was there, spending as much time on it as she was, she was compliant, but as I began giving more time to G. and less to her practices, she agitated to give it up. It was a subtle pressure on me, as if she were saying, 'If Geoffrey is more important than my violin practice, I'll punish you by stopping it.' She knew how exciting I found it to hear her making music with this difficult instrument, and G. was enthusiastic too. He organised a special treat for her after her exam: lunch at the Chinese restaurant. But no: the violin was put aside.

She showed no anxiety, however, when G.M. told the children one day after a meal that G. and I were going to be married. Brigie's reaction was intensely practical. Whereas Jane came round the table and gave me a hug, and Andrew and Michael looked stunned, Brigie said, 'Oh good—that means we'll have three cars in the family.' It was G.'s daughter, Helen, knowing the children better than he did, who realised that Brigie would be the main difficulty in his new family, and it was not long before she found ways of asserting her father's position. Brigie's sharpest sallies were always made in my absence or when I was not in a position to do anything about it. When he and the four of them were together one day she brought out G.M.'s *The Missionaries* from the shelf and made G. read aloud the dedication to me. Much later, after we had moved to our new home and I had gone downstairs one morning, she got into bed with G. and as she settled down said, 'I like this pillow. It smells of Dad.' I confronted her when I heard of these exchanges, and let her know that I understood what she was about: that emotional blackmail was unacceptable (the word itself had to be explained even though she had an instinctive grasp of the concept). I tried to explain to her that her father had chosen to go long before, but as in many other families before and since, the child-mind could not comprehend. Some of her actions were more difficult to confront. On the morning of our marriage, when some of G.'s relatives had joined us, Brigie got out the box of family photographs and entertained the company with a viewing of the pictures of my first wedding. Helen's prediction had proved correct.

There was always this protectiveness towards her father. He had, for her, a slightly romantic aura round him, and he could sense a sexual awareness in her even when she was small. Although they saw him frequently, at weekends and holidays, it must have seemed that he was often away on exotic journeys—to the Sahara, to India, the U.S.A. The fact that he was on television sometimes about his books gave him a certain glamour and her a transferred glory. After G. and I were married, and G.M. had moved back into the Churchfields house, they all saw him more frequently and enjoyed having two houses and the chance for him to share more in their lives.

He took them to France for a fortnight's holiday after G. and I were married and they stayed in a cottage in Brittany. Jane and Andrew were shy about using their school French, and when the milk had to be collected from the farm it was Brigie who said, 'I'll go, Dad. What do I say?', and she would set off down the lane memorising the sentence all the way. She was quite happy, another day, when they were all going for a walk, to stay behind and then go off on her own independent, and probably pre-planned, excursion to the shops.

In the summer after our marriage we moved to Westhill Road on the other side of Hoddesdon. This meant that Jane and Andrew could still attend Sheredes, their comprehensive school, but Brigie and Michael would change junior schools. The school where I taught was still within reach. It was very much like the end of an era: the bulldozers had moved into over-the-back and flattened the magic place to make way for new houses. This first stage was painful, and I was glad to be missing the second. Our new house had its own special qualities and attractions: its mysterious eaves area where children could crawl along under the sloping roof and cob-webs, and storage cupboards under the roof where boys could and did, on the hottest day of the summer, lock them-selves in accidentally. The garden was a private sunny place with tall conifers on either side, and convenient hiding-places behind the rhododendron bushes and Scots pines at the bottom, ideal for the boisterous game of 'run-outs' which was all the rage at the time. There were large gatherings here from time to time when G.'s family and their children came: Celia, Helen and Gareth with Kate, and John and Arja from Sweden with Mark and Robin, the age-range in the two families extending from my father, in his eighties now, to Kate who was born in 1974. They all gathered with other relations for the christening as well.

Here Brigie made new friends, particularly Rebecca next door, and her family, a warm and close-knit group. Brigie loved the company there, Rachel and Anthony, Rebecca's older brother and sister, her father, always ready to joke or tease, and mother, who as well as being good fun, was clever at making things and devising activities, fulfilling many of the functions her own mother did not. Brigie spent as much time next door as she did in her own home, and her diary entries for 1975 and 1976 are full of 'stayed the night at Rebecca's', 'Today I had tea at Rebecca's.' She would join in many of their family activities and went on holiday with them to Northumberland, and appears in many of their family photographs looking as if she belonged. She and Rebecca played wild and naughty games of 'dare' around the houses of the neighbourhood, their nerve amazing and amusing their more dignified older brothers and sisters.

This was one of our favourite games [Rebecca remembers]. We would spend whole evenings sitting on the bonnet of one of the family cars giving each other dares. We'd do such things as knock loudly on the man over the road's garage door when he was working in it and once we even left a lump of fake dog's muck on their doorstep! However, by far and away the most popular dare was to play 'knock down ginger' on the Negus's. We would knock on their door and then run away and hide behind the hedge to watch what happened. By the fourth time in one evening they used to get quite annoyed and come right out to look for us—we used to laugh so much that we thought we'd give ourselves away! If one of us refused to do a dare we had to eat a teaspoonful of salt as a penance. Brigie did this once and spat it over the whole room.

One year at Hallowe'en, Brigie and I decided to go trick or treating. We dressed up in old sheets and carried torches underneath and sacks . . . Mrs. Baker, when she saw us on the front doorstep, said 'Not today thank you,' and shut the door. We spent the whole of the rest of the evening playing knock down ginger on her and generally haunting by tapping on the windows with sticks etc. When it got to the stage of Mrs. Baker chasing us into Cherry Tree Road we decided to call it a day and went home.

Brigie was impressed with Rebecca's small army of guinea pigs and one elderly rabbit called Kip, and there was nothing in the world then that she wanted more than animals of her own. So we constructed a hutch and run at the bottom of the garden and a guinea pig called Huck arrived. It was an eventful time, as Brigie recorded on January 23rd: 'Huck did nine poos on the floor,' and in a month's time, February 22nd, 'Today I got my mineture rabbit a chinchilla one. I am calling it Chile.' The following day, 'I was supposed to go to Anna's but I wanted to stay with my animals.' Rebecca wrote: 'Brigie and I spent a lot of time with our guinea pigs and rabbits. We sometimes undertook great excavations in their runs to make them more interesting for them. We liked to "do" our guinea pigs together, so every morning before school Brigie would come out and yell for me at the top of her voice, which, needless to say, I never failed to hear.'

Brigie's diary records an important event in April: 'Today we put Chile and Kip together. They liked each other and mated.' One day later she observed, rather prematurely we thought, 'Today when I cleaned out my run I notest that Chile was getting fater.' On May 26th: 'Today Chile had her babbys. We think there are four of them. They are sweet.' Alas, Chile proved to be an ill prepared and unloving mother: she must have eaten every one because they simply disappeared. Fortunately Brigie was going to stay with her grandparents and was unaware of the horrible truth.

Her diary records usually petered out in the summer so there is no reference to the early Saturday morning when we all had to rush out in our night clothes and search for Huck.

The Afghan hound from next door had been pulling out the netting from the run and Huck was never seen again. Brigie mourned for him intensely.

Fresh activities opened up in their new school. There was an evening judo club to which Michael and then Brigie were drawn with initial ardent enthusiasm. It certainly looked an appropriate pastime for the rumbustious Michael, but we thought Brigie would hardly be a natural. Great was the clamour to go, however, and Michael was going to be a black belt in no time. Brigie wrote about her progress after the first three or four weeks. February 14th, 'I did my judo grading and got 2 mons.' This notable achievement created a problem: she could not wear these marks of distinction unless she had a suit. Still unconvinced that judo would be a lasting enthusiasm, we had, nevertheless, to get them the gear. Brigie's diary takes up the story. February 28th, 'Today I had judo and fell on my arm and hurt it. There is a big bruse.' March 19th, 'I didn't go to judo because Mummy had a headache.' (That entry did scant justice to the relief she felt.) March 20th, 'Today Mummy said I could leave judo at Easter.' March 21st, 'Today I went to play with Rebecca and Mummy said I could leave judo today.' What a pity, I thought, that the crucial fall had not happened before the suits were bought.

Gymnastics at school proved a longer lasting interest. 'I practised gymnastics in my new laortade on my bed.' 'Today I had gymnastics and passed the hand-stand with bent legs.' 'Geoffrey was impressed at me getting my leg in my arm pit.' And in March 1976, 'Today I was practising gym I can nearly do the splits. Anna had her hair cut yesterday. Mr. Wilson resigned.' The family does not always get a favourable mention at this time. We seem to have given her a rough time in May 1975. On 11th, 'Today Michael slept in my double bed. He is being a pain in the neak.' And on 17th, 'Today Mummy was horrid to me and Michael.'

Even earlier than this, relationships are becoming more important. 'Today the other half of the class went to Mrs.

Powell. I mist Gary,' but six weeks later, however, she feels differently. 'Today I told Anna that I hate Gary.' Her eyes must have been wandering. June 23rd, 'Today Anna didn't come to school. I found out that Stuart loves me 1st.' June 27th, 'Today we went to a silk-worm farm. I kissed Stuart on the back seat.' July 7th, 'Today I went to Hoddesdon to get a badge saying Stuart on.' Six months later, when the new Christmas diary is still an interest, she was writing, 'Today Nathan put his arm round me. I love him.' Although she sent him a Valentine's card, by March 2nd, 'Nathan told me and Anna that he hated us.' There continued to be ups and downs and her friend did not help. 'Today Anna was flirting with Nathan,' but four days later Brigie was reassured: 'Today Nathan told me he likes me. He thinks Anna is a rotten cow.' In spite of all this trauma, other interests remained and in the midst of all this she is recording, 'Today Rebecca gave me some frogsporne.'

Inseparable as Brigie and Rebecca were, they never went to the same school, Brigie joining Jane and Andrew at Sheredes and Rebecca following Rachel to the grammar school in Ware. It is possible that a comprehensive school was not the best place for Brigie. The school had a dedicated young staff who produced their own stimulating and 'enlightened' schemes of work, but I realised that Brigie was always going to be much influenced by her contemporaries. She had undoubted ability but never wanted to stand out for her achievements: the position in the middle was much more to her taste, where she could sink into the background and identify completely with those around her.

It depressed me that she never seemed to allow herself to respond to wider cultural spheres in literature or music. It was as if a positive response to anything for which I or other adults showed enthusiasm was a threat to her position in her own group. G. and I had seen a particularly delightful production of *A Midsummer Night's Dream*: I would take my third years at school, with whom I was reading the play, and also Jane and Brigie. Even the more cynical boys were surprised at how much they enjoyed it. Jane was keen to go and Brigie reluctant. There were other activities which she thought were more compelling, but I told her the story and put my faith in the performance to carry her along. Jane loved it and was sore with laughter at the mechanicals: Brigie sat stony-faced throughout, determined to be impervious. I do remember just the one brief period when she responded to my enthusiasm, sitting rapt and attentive when I was reading aloud some of Walter de la Mare's poetry, and she asked time and again when she was going to bed for a rereading of 'The Listeners'.

She did not keep a diary during the first two years at Sheredes, so her thoughts at the time are unavailable, but the outward signs were worrying. She linked up with the more dissident members of her year group, clamouring to go to the town discos with their doubtful clientele (it was a time when drug-trafficking was reported to be going on in some of the Hoddesdon pubs) and certainly beginning to smoke cigarettes, leaning far out of her bedroom window, as I learned later, to prevent the smell reaching me. She would go off on her perambulations, managing to look tartish even in Jane's borrowed clothes. I was thankful that she was still drawn towards Rebecca, who was not particularly interested in boys at that stage, and very co-operative when she expressed a desire to go to riding lessons with her: it was a healthy antidote, I felt, to the other pseudo-sophisticated activities to which she was drawn. The interest developed apace, and became a major preoccupation. She and Rebecca hardly talked of anything else.

In the summer of 1977 G. and I had a holiday on our own. We took Brigie and Michael to stay with Gladys and Dick and then moved north, stopping in the Dales on the way to Northumberland, which we intended to explore. It rained a great deal there, and after a few days we decided to go back to Yorkshire, as neither of us knew the Dales and the area had looked very inviting. Quite by chance, on yet another wet and bleak Sunday morning, we found a quiet dale that we had not noticed before and stopped at a sign which said 'Morning coffee'. We were treated there with a hospitality the like of which we had never experienced before, and we stayed for the remaining days of our holiday, delighting in the ample meals, the warm log fires, and the grey-green dale with its particular beauty and atmosphere. As we walked along the narrow road one evening, past the post office, G. remarked that he 'would like to run the post office at Litton'.

The dale seemed to us to be the ideal place to live, and G. suggested that the children would love it. We would all come at half-term in October. He was right about their reaction: they responded immediately to the atmosphere and the country, in spite of the fact that we walked them over the hills in driving rain. Brigie for one was very averse to walking: she preferred a horse to do the trudging. But there was always the prospect of Eileen's ample supper at the end of the day, and a long game of Monopoly in front of the fire at night.

G. took John, Mark and Robin to the area in early summer 1978, renting a cottage at Dent, and he enjoyed the week with his son and grandsons. They all came back to Westhill Road and John set off for his work with Swedish children learning English. For a week, before Arja arrived, the boys would be our responsibility. Brigie loved looking after them, especially Robin who was a delightful fair-haired two year old. She was very fond of Mark, too. She had recorded in her diary an incident on the previous Christmas visit: 'Mark sat on my knee and had loads of nuts.' This summer Robin followed her about, lisping her name and holding up his arms to be lifted. It was her first lengthy experience with a young child and she loved it, putting him to bed and changing his nappies even when they were, as John said, 'radioactive'. The little boys even took part in Jane's eighteenth birthday party. It was too exciting to expect them to go to bed. G. had rigged up coloured lights around the garden and there was going to be a barbecue and the Sheredes disco. Brigie helped G. with the drinks from the 'bar' he set up in the hall with the cupboard used for his own daughters' parties years before, and she carried out her role with considerable aplomb. She and I got the boys to bed eventually, and they missed the sight of the dancers performing their rites in rainbow dampness in the garden, under the steady rain that had fallen all evening.

Everything seemed to happen at once that summer. Pompah had been failing fast, and by July had been taken into hospital for 'rehabilitation'; he was to stay there while we had our holiday in Litton. He became very weak, but I was in extreme anxiety that the family should get away. We travelled up to Yorkshire as I knew they would not go without me, but was not surprised when a call came from the hospital on our first morning. I went south again, knowing they were in Eileen's good hands: that original guest house had become almost their second home, and G. would devise some interesting expeditions. I stayed at the hospital for two days and nights, and on the third day the old man's colour changed, his head dropped, there were two deep breaths and he had gone. After two days when the arrangements for his funeral had been made, I went back to Yorkshire and heard all about their activities. Brigie had been riding at Sedbusk, Jane drawing at Arncliffe and Michael finding great riches in a fruit machine at Hawes. The time had been all too short, and we had to get back for Pompah's funeral and school, starting in a few days, but we took a memento, one of Eileen's kittens, a small tabby thing called Freeman (her brothers being Hardy and Willis). We spent the next day tidying the house and cooking for the friends who would come to the funeral, and I suddenly realised that Brigie was very upset. I thought it must be her grandfather's death, even though he was a very old man and she had long since lost contact with him in his confused state. When I asked Brigie, she cried and said, 'I didn't want to leave Yorkshire.' I was surprised at the strength of her feelings. She positively cheered up later, though, at the implications of the funeral the next day.

'Will we be riding in a limousine?' she suddenly asked, and the prospect of this dizzy luxury transformed her gloom.

It was riding of a different sort, on the horses, which was

beginning to fill more of her life. She began writing a diary again in 1979, and reading it is rather like meeting one of John Betjeman's youthful characters.

I rode Zappa today and he was really playing up. He kept walking backwards. At one time I nearly fell off and the reins went right over his head when he jumped . . . We had our private jumping lesson today. I rode Jimmy. Rebecca rode Bubbles. Jimmy kept swerving so we didn't have to jump. Bubbles refused and Rebecca went right over his head . . . We had a hectic ride today. It was boiling. I was wearing a vest top and my arms got really sunburnt. I had to ride Quicky, a twenty-three year old about 12.2 hands who is almost dead. We went to the cornfields at the bottom—the girl on Zappa got frightened because he is very fast in the cornfields. I had to get on Zappa. At the top Jim fell off Kimble and he went running off. Rebecca who was nearest went and caught him. Merry decided to have a roll in the water-splash with his rider still on him.

There were some great rides too. 'We went to the cornfields and cantered down to the second field, which has a great big pond about one foot deep and thirty feet wide and we cantered through it. Then cantered back and we galloped right up the second field. Zappa (I was riding him) was overtaking loads of them. He was really going fast. It's one of my best rides so far.' She started going up to the stables to work at the weekends, one of the small army of horse-mad teenagers who put in long hours for a pittance, in her case from eight thirty until seven thirty for two pounds. That was relatively unimportant to Brigie because she loved being with the horses. On March 24th she recorded,

I got to the stables at eight thirty this morning, brought them all in from the field and groomed Zappa, Fudge and Merry, then I mucked out Rulah's box, Shilo's and Lady's, tacked them up, got everyone on the horses for the ride,

29

untacked them, took them their feeds, had dinner, tacked
them up again, swept the yards, gave them water. Domino
barged past me when I went in his stable and it took ages
to get him in again. He kept kicking. I put rugs on Jimmy,
Luca, Gem and took them out as well as Bubbles, Merry,
Rowan. I was knackered.

At other times the day was fraught as well as tiring. On the
May Day holiday, May 7th,

> I got up to the stable about nine . . . I took Gem out round
> the block to help her leg. Hilary was walking beside me.
> Gem shied twice, the second one she cantered right into
> the middle of the road. In the afternoon, everyone went
> home. I was left to do everything all afternoon. Kimble
> nearly scraped half my thumb off. Lady got scared of being
> tied up. She reared and the rope tightened round my
> finger. I got a blood blister by punching it with a bolt. I got
> another blood blister from somewhere. I couldn't get Blue
> in. I had to do all the feeds for morning and night. I was
> really cross, so was Mum.

It was far too much responsibility for a thirteen-year-old.
    Even though she was earning very little for all this work,
she had her finances worked out in detail. On May 15th she
writes,

> I have worked out that by July (when the French come) I
> will have thirty-five pounds. I know that if I get the
> vacuum cleaner, the T-shirt, the other white top, the
> double V-neck, the straight skirt, the pink blouse and my
> ears pierced it will all come to £34 and 4p. So I will just
> have enough. After that I want a Bikini and some Jodhpurs
> (brown). Ray Brazier asked me out today. I said no. I am
> knackered. My sunburn is killing me. I fancy Gary who
> owns Jacy or Mr. J.B. He's a laugh. He is fifteen. Hey good
> looking (that's an advert). I'm in a funny mood.

That mood was dampened the next day, unfortunately.

I have had a row with Mum, so she won't let me take Rebecca's bike to the stables. She said I have got to mend the puncture Michael made (he denies it) again. I have already done it once but it didn't work. I can't do it because the pump has been lost so I have got to buy a new one with my money so that has cocked up my plans for clothes. I will have to work extra at the stables, or not get one of the tops. SHIT.

But she did buy our present, the vacuum cleaner, a small gadget for the car. She had already been to France in April on an exchange visit, and a long list of clothes had been made for that too. She stayed at Marcigny with Lisa, whom she liked, and she recorded some of the things they did. 'We went to Vichy. It is where the water is made that is very good for your kidneys. This evening my family went to church. I went to Sally's. We drank champagne to celebrate Easter.' She was very impressed with a French riding school that they went to, and then there was a fair. 'Sally went off with Didier and I went off with Gérard. Lisa went off with a girl she knew. After we went to the cafe and had a coke.' She felt ill the next day and couldn't go to the stadium with Gérard, but he came to see her. 'He was really comforting and when I was with him I felt much better.' Judging by the subsequent diary entries, most of her impressions of France related to Gérard and his promise to come and see her in England.

This is in contrast to the rest of her diary for the third year at Sheredes, which is much less concerned with boys than the previous ones. There are occasional references to being asked to go out, but the offers are invariably refused. The boys she 'fancied' were all much older, and there is a tone of resignation in her comments. 'I still want to go out with David in the sixth year, but I'm sure he doesn't like me.' 'None of the boys I like would go out with me.' Elaine had become her great friend at school, and it is her relationships that Brigie speculates on with interest. 'Laine doesn't want to go out with him but he walks her home and goes round to her house but she doesn't want him to. He hasn't asked her out yet but I think he will.' 'F. has chucked Laine. She phoned me . . . and she told me all about it. He said it was because they were in a routine, and she said to me a few days ago that's what would break them up.' Some of her remarks about the boys are scathing: 'M.B. gets slimier every day (a bit like J.R. on *Dallas*)', and of another boy, 'I really hate him. The only word I can describe him as is Pukey.'

We had some important news to give her when she came back from France. About six months before we had suddenly realised that there was nothing to stop us fulfilling a long-felt desire to move away from the London area. Until we found Littondale there had never been a particular place which felt sufficiently compelling. Now the place and the time con-verged. Jane had finished school, Brigie and Michael had not yet started their O level courses, Andrew would be happy to stay with G.M. and finish his A levels at Sheredes, and G. came to an arrangement with the *Guardian* to do some of his writing from home. For months we had studied all the estate agents' sheets and the local papers of the area, and Eileen was on the look-out for houses. Nothing suitable appeared and finally G. and I decided to comb the area in the February half-term. We started at Richmond, trying to persuade ourselves that there were other dales equal in quality to Littondale. If we had found a house, no doubt we could have made that mental leap, but there was nothing, and as we came up the road to Eileen's it was just like coming home. If all else failed we would take a rented house in Arncliffe while we searched the following year. Eileen knew of no houses likely to come on the market, and we went to Skipton the next day, Friday, and bought the *Craven Herald*. The selection on the lists seemed just as it had been for weeks and G. returned to his coffee and some other reading matter. I was still glancing casually at the page when I spotted an obscure amateur advertisement and showed it to him. The telephone number startled him. 'That's Litton Post Office!' he said, and we rushed out to confirm it at the nearest telephone box. He was right, and we spent the rest of the day going back and forth through the floods at Kilnsey trying to make contact with the postmaster, Mr. Battersby. We were the first of the many would-be buyers to see the house that night and we made the owner an offer. He was not ready to commit himself and we had to leave the next morning in total uncertainty about our prospects.

All the way south I imagined the family's reaction to the news that we had made an offer for that house. I remember one thing about our phone call to them at G.M.'s when we got back: they were all very excited, but most vivid was the controlled and vibrant excitement in Brigie's voice, 'It sounds good, Mum!' The following weeks were very tense: we all wanted that house very badly, and as the delay went on and we heard it was going to be auctioned (under its private name of Barn Garth House) at some date painfully distant, we wrote Mr. Battersby a letter stressing our concern to keep the post office going and we made an improved offer. Easter Sunday that year was memorable: Freeman had her first kittens and Mr. Battersby rang up. 'By and large,' he said, he was accepting our offer. We were not quite sure what that meant, but the statement seemed to justify some of the wild rejoicing that followed, even though G. cautioned that a more guarded optimism would be wiser. That was the news we had to give Brigie on her return from France. 'Mum was waiting for me,' she wrote, 'and she said Freeman had got five kittens and we are probably going to get Litton Post Office.'

That was how we came to buy our house in Yorkshire and many were the hours we spent visualising it to each other and making delightful plans for our move. We came up in May so that Brigie could take her tests at the Girls' High School. For me it was like going back to my old New Zealand school of thirty years before: the dignified portraits of previous head-mistresses lining the staircase, the racks of indoor shoes neatly under the navy-blue garments. For Brigie the contrast with Sheredes could not have been stronger: this quietly formal atmosphere where gowns and mortar-boards, one felt, would not have been out of place. It was an uncomfortable day for her, coping with a positively streaming cold. She gives an account in her diary.

We went to Skipton and bought some hankies and a Vicks inhaler for me. We got to the girls' school at nine thirty. I met the headmistress, then Mum went. I started off doing one English exam. It was quite hard. I had to do it in the gym on my own. I felt very ill. My next exam was French. It was very difficult. Some girls took me round the school at break. At dinner break they took me into dinner. It was sausages, chips, then ice cream. After dinner I had another English, then maths. They were both quite easy.

The rest of the day was more enjoyable.

When we got home we went to Mr. Battersby's house (ours to come) to see the post office. It is really lovely. It has lots of little gadgets, like a door that slides upwards, a shutter in a wall so the telephone can go into two rooms. It has a very nice garden. [The next day] We went and served in the post office, about ten people came in. I served quite a lot of them, because Mum came round and we all had coffee in the kitchen and I didn't mind serving the people who came in then.

Much as she wanted to live in Litton there were some aspects of the move which were painful. On July 20th, 'It was sad to-day. Elaine had brought a lovely big card saying sorry you're leaving. Everyone in my group and some other friends had signed it.' Elaine was an important friend and she hoped 'that Helen and Elaine will go round together when I leave'. For Zappa at the stables, she had a special feeling, and I remember that one day when I went to collect her, she was standing motionless leaning against him, her arms round his neck, bracing herself for the parting. It was going to be hard to leave G.M. too. All this time she had been able to see him and her diary is full of references: 'Today I went to Daddy's and Barbara's. I helped Daddy in the garden. It was very nice.'

Brigie was upset and worried about his loneliness after the break-up of his second marriage, and she would go to see him after school from Sheredes. Marilyn has spoken about the serious appraisal and detailed questioning that she received from Brigie when she first entered their lives later on. Brigie must have wanted to assure herself that this was a fit person to be with her father, and Marilyn obviously passed that test because they became good friends and Brigie would share many of her experiences with Marilyn on a more equal basis than she could with me. When they acquired Sam, a boisterous Labrador, there were eventful walks. 'We had quite a long walk today. Sam went off with another dog and Marilyn couldn't get him back. He went right on to the road. . . . I phoned up Marilyn to say happy birthday to Sam and she had forgotten it.' There were horse activities too: 'Marilyn and I went riding today. She was not allowed to have a ride because they didn't know how good she was, so we both had a lesson. She rode Gem. She is quite good, although I think she's forgotten a lot.' In March she is relieved that G.M.'s book got a good review. It was good to have another house to go to: 'I went to Dad's for dinner with Elaine because we are not allowed in school because the teachers are on strick at dinner times.' He was becoming more of a real person for her now that the contact was more casual and informal and they could see him whenever they pleased. She would challenge him when she thought he was being too critical of other people and comment later if she felt he was being 'soppy'. They all had a barge holiday together after we left Westhill Road. After telling the tales of how various people and Sam fell in, Brigie says: 'I can't wait to go to Litton but I don't want the holiday to end.' After taking the boat back they spent another night at Churchfields. 'Dad took me to Broxbourne Station. We said goodbye to Marilyn, Sam and Andrew. I just about held off my tears. It was really horrid when Dad said goodbye. I had tears in my eyes he could see. When the train pulled out and Dad was out of sight I burst out crying. We travelled up on the 125. Yorkshire was sunny and Barn Garth House is lovely . . .'

# 2

*Litton*

It was a time of high excitement as they realised they were actually living here now, not just coming for fleeting visits. There was everything to do and to explore: difficult for them to know where to start, especially as we knew only a few people in the village at the beginning. Brigie saw herself behind the counter in the shop, arranging the Mars bars and the Mintoes, being brisk and efficient. It was disillusioning, though, to sit there for half an hour waiting for the next customer. 'Come on all you people,' she said to the air once in exasperation, 'come and buy our lovely things.' So her career as a Litton shopkeeper was short-lived, and she was off to the farm instead, a much more exciting place. Stewart would be there, like the Pied Piper, with a troop of children following him about, chattering away to them, making jokes, letting them help. Brigie and Michael soon joined in.

She developed a sense of hearing for tractors: sitting in the kitchen she would cock her ear. 'Tractor!' she would shout, grab a jacket and fly. Stewart, or Stephen, would obligingly stop for her to climb on, and she would join the crowd sitting in the trailer or standing on the rickety vehicle, looking as if she had been travelling that way for years. There was the last of the hay-making to be done, and they learned to heave the heavy bales into the barns, to help get the cows in for milking, to wash the bottles and help with the milk-round. They spent hours at the farm: it was another over-the-back but more spacious, and definitely a real world rather than make-believe. Here it was urgent that the hay was got for the winter feed, and sometimes animals actually died. They came back with tales of cows with mastitis or milk fever, full of the horrific detail that Stewart loved to give them, and they shared in the tension when a calf was ill and the vet called in.

Brigie wrote about the farm activities in her diary:

Michael drove the tractor today. He felt really pleased with himself. I hope I can . . . I went to Spittle. Stewart was walling and the rest of us went to teach me to drive the tractor. The trouble was that they couldn't get it to go, so I didn't have a go. Stewart drove us back, with us on the back in the transport box . . . I had a real day today (real = good, great in Yorkshire) . . . After dinner Michael and I went to the sheep dipping with Stewart and Stephen. It was good fun. I helped hold them, while Stewart cut off the wool round their tails, for tupping time.

This was in October: in November,

Michael, Colin [Eileen's husband], Stephen and I went up on the hillside to try and kill a rabbit. We weren't allowed to talk and Colin shone the flashlight for Stephen to shoot when he saw a rabbit. Stephen went off up the hill on his own, Michael went back, and Colin and I waited at the top of their croft. We heard a gun fire and Colin thought he saw a rabbit running away. Stephen came back, mad 'cos he hadn't got one, then he held an enormous one up. Colin gutted it, which made me feel sick . . . Michael shot four rats with the gun that Colin has lent him.

After their evening meal, it was always 'Can we go to Eileen's?'—just across the road—and they would sit in her kitchen, listening to stories of the farm and the lore of the area, soaking it all up, putting down their roots in this new

38

home. Brigie loved the verbal sparring that she got there with Colin and Stephen, sharp and perky banter flying about. She could say anything to Colin, Eileen said. She had an answer for everything, and he relished it. He said later he came to regard Brigie as a daughter. About that time, Brigie wrote, 'Stephen kept making fun of me. Colin made me drink a mug of this revolting lemon drink for my cold because I felt worse.' I was worried that she might be outstaying her welcome and becoming cheeky, but instead they were disappointed if she did not turn up. She and Stephen became good friends: he did not have Stewart's easygoing tolerance for hordes of children but liked seeing them singly. He was quieter than his brother, but thoughtful too, and he and Brigie were sharp partners in good-natured gibes: they understood each other, Eileen said. Later when Jane and Stephen fell in love, Brigie, I sensed, was rather put out, although she never commented.

A major reason for Brigie's enthusiasm for living in the Dales was the glittering prospect, as she saw it, of having her own horse. Nothing had ever been promised but obviously there was more prospect here than in the suburbs of Hoddesdon. One of the first things she did here was to make a survey of the horses in the village. The most intriguing combination was a brown Dales pony carrying a girl with white spiky punk-rock hair, an incongruous sight in this small remote village, and Brigie's contact with the person under the hair was at first a bit tentative. This was Alison, staying with Janet and her daughter, Katie, at Armisteads Farm and recovering from an abortive sixth-form course in London. She became a very good friend to Brigie, who respected her knowledge about horses and liked her intelligence and pungency. They would ride together up the old road and let the horses gallop on the splendid flat part at the top, Brigie on Helen, the Dales pony, and Alison on Eileen's Tosca, who was more than Brigie could manage. On September 2nd Brigie wrote, 'I had the most brilliant ride today. I rode Helen, Katie rode Andy, and Alison rode Tosca. We went up the Stainforth track. We went seven

39

miles and for at least four of them we galloped and cantered. Helen was really good. When we got back I gave her a good groom.' Alison soon began to look more in keeping with the landscape: the punk style disappeared, and she donned the gear of a Yorkshire farm girl, with heavy man's overcoat and enormous wellingtons. This was where the contrast in their attitudes was most obvious, Brigie being very fastidious about her appearance at all times. But she never commented about this, even when they travelled to London together some months later, Alison still in the attire of her outdoor life up here. Time was when Brigie would have been highly embarrassed at this unconventional behaviour.

All too soon the new-found freedom had to be interrupted with a trip to Skipton to buy school clothes. It was going to be a shock to Brigie to don the staid outfit of the High School after the smart and colourful uniform of Sheredes. She was resigned in theory and was moderately acquiescent about the blazer. Plain white blouses and a tie were accepted with considerable reluctance, but when it came to trying on a navy-blue winter coat her limited tolerance was exhausted.

'I'm not going to wear a thing like that! It makes me look about fifty!' Jane and I pointed out that everyone else would be wearing them and that she would freeze without it. Brigie described it in her diary, 'A coat which is really horrid but it will be warm. I was a bit agged because I had to get that coat.' We bought her a smart striped T-shirt to restore morale, and then she cheered up, remembering that I had promised to let her have her way with shoes in the fourth year. Later on she chose a pair to her taste and I tried not to look at them. She recorded the event: 'I was dreading buying new shoes. I tried on a pair that were quite high after a bit of persuading, but Mum thought they were too tight. I tried another pair on which were three and a half inch heels and after a big row Mum let me have them. So hooray my first pair of high shoes.' When she first wore them to school, though, 'It was embarrassing because I didn't think I could walk in them.'

She envied Michael, who did not need uniform at Upper Wharfedale, and it was a great effort, much resented, to put on the tie that first morning. I suppose she was nervous about going, but she did not show it, and set off with Margaret Walker and her daughters to catch the bus at Lane End. Luckily there was another new girl, Joanne, in her form and they quickly became friends. As the weeks went by more names were mentioned and they were obviously joining in a group. Life in the form room was fun with one or two slightly mad colleagues, who without being rebels were lively and refreshing. We have photos that she took of them all in their room at school, friendly, open girls, ready to giggle at authority, warm-hearted and very loyal to each other.

The Girls' High School was a good experience for Brigie, although she resented the rules and what seemed to her like the pettiness of a very traditional establishment. Quite early on, her earrings, two in each ear, came under the close scrutiny of the headmistress Miss Kent, and letters on the subject were exchanged between school and home. She objected fiercely to what she saw as the unfairness of it as other girls, she said, were wearing more earrings than she was with impunity. She devised means of coping with the situation, one of which was to remove the offensive adornments before the R.E. lesson with Miss Kent. The school was, however, able to do something for her which Sheredes, for all its idealism, had not. Here she was surrounded by friends whose parents were concerned about their education, and for all the fun they had together there was an underlying seriousness about work or, at the very least, a dread of the consequences if they had a bad report.

Although the work at Skipton was often boring, exercise books being filled with notes taken from dictation, she made less fuss about this than about the restrictions which impinged on her freedom more obviously: the earrings issue and the necessity of taking a note every time she wanted to go to 'town' at lunch time. These times were numerous as they were an opportunity to see the Ermysteds boys and pick up the latest gossip about who was 'going out' with whom, and there had to be some small item of shopping to provide the excuse. She was feeling some frustration by the beginning of November. 'Instead of having games at Sandylands we had to spend two lessons cleaning the tops of our desks with Vim and Brillo pads. It was really boring. We had to do it because someone had been writing "rude and crude remarks" on the desks. I got splattered with Vim, it went all over my skirt. There is a disco on at Gargrave tonight. I really wanted to go. I'm sick of staying home listening to people talking about their boyfriends.' Two days later, 'I've got no one who fancies me. I really want to go out with someone again and go to some discos and have lots of clothes. I can't go to discos easily though, partly 'cos I live so far away and partly 'cos I've got no one to go with. It's very depressing.' Four days later there was another cri de coeur, 'I want a boyfriend. I haven't been out with a lad for ages and ages and ages and ages and ages and ages.' In a fortnight, though, Joanne is asking her to stay the night and go with a group to the ice-skating in Bradford.

Wider horizons began to open up, parties and discos in Skipton when she stayed the night with Joanne, and the local discos here when Joanne would come back with her. Even higher heels were produced for these occasions. 'Well, you did say I could choose my own shoes in the fourth year!' There was one night in early winter, with snow falling, when the two young ladies, shrieking and giggling, teetered and slithered out to the car, their ludicrous sandals totally out of place with the conditions. Glamour was all, though, and the eye-shadows and lip-shiners as well were amazing to behold. Even more amazing was the sight of Brigie when I trailed down to collect her at 12 p.m., as often as not outside the hall in a passionate embrace with some youth, oblivious to the flashing lights and blaring music within. The youngest daughter was growing up fast.

The first time a pub disco was yearned for I vetoed the idea, much to Brigie's annoyance, but when I realised later that everyone else was going to these events it seemed un-realistic and she went, with an accompanying warning about drinking. 'Oh, Mum, we know what we're doing, you know. You don't need to tell me!' Even so, it emerged that at one party Martini had nearly been her undoing.

Some of the boys became names instead of shadowy figures at the doorway of a disco. One glorious and unattainable youth was the head boy of Ermysteds, no less, who sent her enigmatic and tantalising messages through a go-between, but she soon realised that she did not have a chance with him and accepted her fate with grace. The arrangements and rearrangements of who was 'going out' with whom, among the pupils of the two schools in Skipton, became too com-plicated and fast-moving for me to keep up with, but by the time they were in the fifth year the 'going out' seemed to last longer. The term itself, it occurred to me, was something of a misnomer as the transporting there and back was invariably done by us, and I had many opportunities as I waited outside a disco on a cold winter's night to reflect somewhat ironically on the semantics.

When she was not going out at the weekend it was always good fun to help at Eileen's, and often during the week as well. She liked it when there were a number of guests to be served dinner at night, and would even leap out of bed unwontedly early on a Saturday to help with breakfasts. Eileen found her quick and useful in the routine. With one group particularly, several R.A.F. officers leading a survival course in the area, she became very friendly: they liked her quick, bright manner and she enjoyed their teasing jokes. They told her she could be a 'casualty' for them, lying prone on the moors to be rescued by their pupils. It would mean missing school and she knew I would not agree, so they composed a joke letter that she brought home. It was addressed 'Dear Teacher' and asked for Brigie's essential services. It was signed 'Francis Pym'. Even if I had given in I doubt whether she would actually have enjoyed lying on a cold moor, even in somewhat glamorous circumstances, hating cold and wet as much as she did. To compensate for her disappointment they promised her a ride in a helicopter when they came up later, and a large bunch of flowers arrived for her after they had left. They came several times after that, and it was Dave among them who was her special friend. He loved riding too, and he told her about the Arab horses he had ridden in southern Arabia when he served there. He was here, too, at the beginning of the historic snowfall of April 24th, 1981, a week after a blazing Easter, when he found the conditions too real even for them, and took his trainees home again. Brigie went with G. that afternoon through the snow to collect his father at Skipton. It was an eventful journey there and back, most notably when they did a 360-degree skid at Rylstone. We had eighteen inches of snow that day, the power went off, and Andrew, Brigie and Michael worked till midnight, helping Stephen and Stewart to milk the cows by hand. Brigie went to bed after that, but the others were up most of the night helping with the lambing.

By about the end of our first winter here G. suggested that we should seriously think of getting Brigie a horse. She was ecstatic about the prospect and had long consultations with Eileen's friend, Bob. By early July he had found an eight-year-old chestnut mare: he had known the horse nearly all her life and she was a lively ride, he said, but very good-tempered. We went over to Ingleton to see her. She stood, tall and beautiful, with her fully grown foal in the yard of the farm, her ears pricked and alert. Brigie had trouble mounting her as she was so high, and the rider looked small on the horse as they went off down the fields, but Brigie seemed to be at ease. Apart from one hesitation, the horse was doing as she wanted. We all liked the look of Shez very much, and were even more impressed to hear that her registered name was Bishop's Prayer and that she actually had a passport as well. With all this dignity and spirit the only question was whether Brigie could manage her. She soon decided, though, and Bob would bring her over in his wagon. Dennis, a neighbouring farmer, in spite of his aversion to horses, offered grazing on his hill field, the Brow. It was a pity that Alison had gone back to London and could not share that early excitement.

Brigie was intensely happy, but nervous as well, and the first rides were modest affairs, simply round the outgang, which must have been a bit tame for Shez, used as she was to gathering sheep on Ingleborough. Sensing Brigie's uncertainty, she started refusing her orders, and Brigie had quite a tussle to get the mastery of her, but there were some great rides before the roads became too slippery in the winter. G. and I came upon them once on the road from Arncliffe in the deep twilight: it was too dark for them to be out, but Brigie was high with ecstasy.

'This is the best day yet!' and I could tell that she heard not a word of our warning. However, there were frightening moments too: one day on Barks, the hill down to Halton Gill from the Pen-y-Ghent road, Shez 'took off' and Brigie just had to hang on. 'It was really scary,' she said.

Alison came up later for a week or two, and she loved riding Shez. She and Brigie would go off together up the old road. Alison wrote about it later:

She could fly up the hills hardly sweating and with such a delicate action that her hooves seemed to almost fly with her. Yet it was when she galloped that Brigie and I found her true strength and I will never forget that feeling. Brigie and I loved Shez's gallop best. To gallop on Shez was to feel her powerful quarters gather underneath and then spring, releasing such sheer strength that the first spring took your breath as a great gush of wind flew in your face.

Brigie would have appreciated that description, but I think she got equal pleasure from looking after Shez in the winter.

She started working on Saturdays at the gift shop in Skipton, and a large part of her earnings went towards equipping and feeding Shez. She bought a New Zealand rug for her when the weather got cold and contributed half the cost of hay and winter feed. Her requested Christmas present that year from G.M. and Marilyn was an indoor rug for Shez. Stephen and Stewart had offered a loose-box at the farm to house her, and Stephen and Andrew constructed a stable door. She and sometimes Robyn, her young friend, were down there every night after school, mucking her out and talking to her. 'I tell her all my secrets, you know,' she said to me later. Sometimes she would get up early to take her across the river to the Brow, before school when the weather was fit, but sometimes if the ford was flooded or Brigie had overslept, that duty fell to me. Although I complained, it was good to handle that splendid creature and compensate for my own childhood longing for a horse. Brigie took the care of Shez very seriously and was deeply hurt if anyone suggested that she was not doing right by her. At these times it was as if a mother was being criticised for lack of care for her baby.

What with Shez and school and boyfriends, it was a busy life. Sometimes it was a visitor to the village who became her passion, like John from Huddersfield, and she was flattered by the attention of Neil who came for the clipping. The ancient school bus, lumbering on its slow journey to Skipton, was a useful meeting-place, and I think it was here that she got to know Gumby, for whom she had a wild, if brief, infatuation. He was much in demand, it seemed, and she regarded it as a matter of great pride that she was 'going out' with him for longer than any of his previous girlfriends. But towards the end of a breathtaking two months he became silent and moody on the bus, and finally she could no longer pretend that it was just the worry of his A levels. One day the telephone call came to say that it was ended. She sat down miserably in the kitchen, and I tried consoling remarks. 'Oh well, I knew he'd finish with me—I knew he would!' and she laughed. She was hurt, but she went off down to the farm to think about other things, and probably talk to Shez about it.

James was another friend on the bus. He was always asking her to 'go out' with him, but she resisted. He must have been very patient because he kept returning to the subject. One incident that she related then came to mind later in very different circumstances. The elderly bus often broke down, but there was one spectacular incident when, as Brigie described it, the bus 'blew up'. She and James were sitting at the back when there was a loud bang and a heavy bolt flew off the floor, just missing them both. Smoke came through and Brigie leapt down the aisle, the first to reach the safety of the roadside. 'Just think,' James said to her afterwards, 'we might have been killed and then perhaps you would have gone out with me in heaven.'

By now Brigie was well established in her new environment and so was Michael. Their interests had taken them on different courses, Brigie to her horse and her social life, and Michael to his gamekeeping, but there was a strong bond. The rather unequal relationship of the early school years, when Michael had depended on Brigie for advice, had changed into a real friendship, and they were much together, watching television up in his room, Brigie painting her fingernails while she sat there, sharing complaints about the rest of us, going off together to the farm, where he joined in more of the work than she did. She would beg him to wait for her while she donned all her garments, hating to be cold, and he would stand there with good-natured impatience, scoffing in his new toughness at her 'feeble' ways. He could give *her* advice now, moving rapidly as he was into the men's world up here. Theirs was the closest friendship in the family.

Between Jane and Brigie the earlier tensions remained, increased now by the fact that they had to share a bedroom, as the boys did. Brigie had it to herself during term time, and when Jane came home from art school for the holidays, spreading her clothes (all bought at the Oxfam shop) around the small space, Brigie looked very askance, and even more when Jane put them on. They were so different: Brigie with her fastidiousness and Jane with her unconventional and seeming carelessness about her appearance. Whereas Brigie would carry her small hairbrush everywhere she went, concerned to keep her long and curly hair in good order, Jane would sometimes not touch hers till midday or later. Brigie's mind was full of the current boyfriend, or the one on the horizon, and the next disco, and Jane was preoccupied with her art work. Even so, she could sometimes look on Brigie with an amused tolerance, in spite of the irritations, and was able to take her part. When I was upset at Brigie's rejection of one boyfriend for whom I felt a good deal of sympathy, Jane explained, 'Well, she just wants to play the field. It's all right, everybody does.'

Andrew was here all through our second year in Litton, and as events turned out this was very fortunate. Brigie and Andrew had an affinity: there was not the underlying rivalry as there was with her sister. She would accept his teasings and gibes, and she liked him because he was tall and good-looking and he was her older brother. They were more akin in appearance: Jane and Michael have a roundness from Gladys and from me and Brigie and Andrew the more sharply defined features of their father. They were the middle two of the family, and they had settled into an easy and accepted familiarity. With the four of them, there was always the feeling of a group: they always remembered each other's birthdays, wanted to know how each was faring and had a sense of solidarity. It is strange, looking back to Brigie's last winter with us, to remember how many evenings there were when they were all sitting round the fire, and the talk would go back to the early days and 'Do you remember when . . . ?' There were memories of over-the-back and friends there, tales about school and daring adventures that I had not known about. It was almost as if they were summing up their joint childhood, recording and exploring it before they went their separate ways.

Brigie had long ago decided that *she* would not go to university—all that *effort*!—but she would get a job, like brucellosis testing, which would take her round to different farms. I think she saw this as a chance to meet some young, rich farmer who would indulge her taste for clothes and horses. To this end, she battled with her biology, finding it very hard. She would take it on to A level, with English and geography.

I had wondered earlier how she would cope with the traditional Eng Lit course, never having read any Shakespeare or serious novels, and my heart sank when she said *Northanger Abbey* was her set book. She would be too young for it, I thought, and prepared a defence against dismissive comments. Fortunately I was wrong; she developed very much in her final year, and the book, judging by an essay she wrote at the end of her course, led her to a new self-awareness which seemed to me the beginning of a real response to literature.

I have quite frequently heard it said [she wrote], that *Northanger Abbey* is best read at a slightly later stage in life than we have read it and it is a pity for those who didn't get any enjoyment out of the book, possibly because they were too young to appreciate it properly, because they might well have been totally 'put off' the rest of Jane Austen's works after this one. Henry Tilney, although just a figment of the imagination, has helped me. He has made me conscious of those childish, immature aspects of Catherine's character, which are vaguely similar to mine in some ways. It also made me realise that everyone is like Catherine Morland at some point in their lives because just like she read novels like *Udolpho* which aided her growing-up, we nowadays read books like *Northanger Abbey*! It is obvious that we are going through the same sort of process as she was at this stage in her life. Whether this is the reason that this type of book is set or not, I don't know, but it certainly helped me to discover some of my childish and immature attitudes and ideas, and it makes me want to alter them, so as not to appear as inexperienced and silly as Catherine did.

Three months later, as the time for O level results came nearer, she was nervous. She rang me from Skipton to tell me, very pleased, that she had an 'A' for literature and 'B' for language, 'C' for geography and, even more gratifying, a 'C' for biology. She had failed history and physical science, as she expected, having concentrated on her proposed A level subjects. How like Brigie it was to have achieved just what she needed, and with no 'wasted' effort.

All through this time she was becoming more com-panionable in many ways, chattering away about events at school, clothes she wanted to buy, funny things at the farm, the boyfriends (of one nameless youth, 'He's really thick, you know, Mum!'). At five fifteen on a school day when the door flew open and there was a loud 'Hi!' to let us know it was not a customer, there would always be something interesting to tell or some outrage to be mollified. Life with Brigie was never dull. She often thought me very unreasonable when I refused her some plan, and would go into a silent fury, hoping to make me relent. If the denial was final, however, she could accept defeat with a good grace. She told me what her friends thought about it. 'Your Mum's really strict with you, isn't she? She doesn't look as if she is but she's really strict!' There was no accusation in this, just an acceptance that there were limits. I think she needed these, but it meant, I realised later, that there were things she could not tell me. Mary Ann said that she would go into the gift shop on a Saturday morning sometimes and announce, 'I've just had a row with Mum, and she won as usual.' I did not always win, however, and sometimes found it difficult to deal with this daughter who was so different from Jane, and from me as well. We could laugh at each other a good deal, and she would have some sharp sallies at my self-importance or other illusions of grandeur, and go off with the gay, mocking laugh that was half affection and half emphasis of the point she had made.

I had given up trying to coax her against her will into theatre visits, for instance, or church-going. The lip would curl and I would know it was a lost cause. Sometimes I tried to bridge the gap between what I felt and what she seemed to assume. When I was going to church, she would say, 'Have a nice time,' not in a mocking way, but in the conviction that nobody in their right mind would go anywhere without that prospect. Once I got back, and she said, 'Did you have a nice time?' and I struggled for words to explain the challenge and commitment of worship. There was a silence while I considered.

'Well, why do you go if you don't enjoy it?' she asked impatiently.

'It's not that sort of enjoyment.'

In the end she was the one to find a word. 'Well, was it satisfying then?'

'Yes, it was. That's much better.' The point settled, she went off on her own much more comprehensible pursuits.

She was always glad that we had come to live in Litton, envying me that I could stay here all day, when she had to go to school, not that she wanted me to go back to work. 'I don't want you to go teaching again. You laugh much more since we've been up here.' She was never demonstrative with affection and retreated from displays of emotion. In keeping with her age she was often thoughtless and careless, but now and again there would be a sudden, surprising recognition of some small service performed for her. 'You're really good to us, Mum. We don't take enough notice, but you're really good.'

G. received the same recognition sometimes for his thoughtfulness to me, or to her. When he bought electric blankets for them on the first cold night up here, or got a heater for her bedroom, and the day we came home with a sheepskin jacket he had got for my birthday, 'Oh, that's really nice, Geoffrey!' she said with strong emphasis. Her connection with him had grown considerably since the early ambivalent times, although she still had it in her power to irritate him extremely or to delight him extremely. Even when he was tired of trailing down the dale to collect her from the bus, he was always glad to see her; she was such bright and lively company and she impressed him with her sensitivity to the beauty of our surroundings. The dale, he felt, would never be the same without her. Her diary records,

51

'Geoffrey took me to school today because he was going shopping. He bought Michael and I an electric blanket each, they are really lovely and warm. I have started having blankets as well as a duvay because winter is setting in and I was cold last night. There is snow on Pen-y-Ghent and on the tops of the hills of our lovely dale.' He, too, produced strong reactions in her: she could not understand the pressures of his work and was not tolerant of the tension they sometimes caused in him, but she delighted in his wit, and the hilarious but deadpan exaggerations in which he excelled.

Coming to Litton had been a joint adventure for the whole group, a cementing together, with new shared experiences and qualities emerging in members of the family that some of us had not seen before. These perhaps would have become apparent in the natural process of maturing, in time spent together, but the new environment and the fresh focus made it more obvious. The place itself with all our individual reactions to it made it an important part of the family story.

If Brigie knows about me writing this, she might well respond to those last sentences with the remark she made once when I meditated aloud on the effects of changing one's life from the busyness and bells of school to the quiet and gentle routine of a country post office. I was thinking aloud about the challenge of infinite available time and its sometimes frightening prospect.

'Goodness,' she said to the others with a laugh, 'I've never seen her go on like this before. She's getting quite philosophical.'

Brigie herself had no time for 'philosophy', particularly in the summer of 1981. She could not wait, as she said, for the exams to be over, and the exercise books thrown out. (I surreptitiously kept some in case she needed to repeat biology, at least.) She had suddenly become friends with Kate at the pub, and they planned a celebratory week camping with their horses at the Dagetts' farm at Burnsall. It was strange that she and Kate had stayed aloof up until this stage: they were in the same year at school, both had horses, and both lived in Litton. But something suddenly clicked and Brigie often went down to see Kate at night, and helped her father, Steve, in the bar on Bank Holidays. She was busy there at Easter, making sandwiches with Kate, and even pulling pints.

They talked about their holiday for weeks, and the giggling and shrieking that went on during the planning sessions made us less than confident that they would cope with the practicalities. They finally got off one Monday morning, riding the horses, while Val, Kate's mother, took the tent and gear by car. It was a marvellous week; the whole Dagett family became involved with their escapades, Nigger and Sparky (otherwise Nigel and Michael), who were contemporaries at Ermysteds, helping with the tent and any other daunting problems, and meals seemed to have been alternately camp-style meals for the lads, or Margaret Dagett's undoubtedly better organised indoor ones for Brigie and Kate. It was a week of great fun and happiness and they could not stop talking about it after they rode back on Friday. The next morning, when I drove them to collect their tent, I soon realised what a warm and hospitable family it was, and could understand the girls' enthusiasm. Margaret and I would meet again, we decided, and she would bring her daughter Helen up to Litton to see where these older and slightly crazy girls lived. Brigie and Kate would go back there at Christmas to help with the turkey-plucking.

Brigie had thought she would be working full-time at the gift shop but this did not happen as business was quiet, and so there was a lull in the holiday. In July, Steve planned to snatch a few days from the pub and invited Brigie to go with him and Kate to Scotland. That was another exciting prospect. On July 2nd she finally decided to go to the doctor about a swelling on her left hand between the finger and the thumb. He said it was a ganglion, as we had thought, and that it would either go away itself or she could bang it with a heavy book, like a bible. She thought, for the time being anyway, she would take the former option. My cousin Helen and her daughter Moira came down for a few days from Edinburgh on July 13th, and Helen remembers that although she was teaching Brigie to tat she did not notice the swelling, in spite of her medical training. Brigie and Moira went off to help with the hay-timing, as it is called in Litton, and came back tired after lifting the bales. Brigie and Kate set off for Scotland on July 20th, Steve driving through the night to Dornock. They had a great time there too, and came back full of tales about the huge meals, the midnight swimming, and interesting 'encounters'. They were no sooner back than they were off again, this time to Broxbourne to stay with G.M. and Marilyn during the Royal Wedding week, but they seemed not to have taken much notice of that, being more interested in the London shops. They saw Rebecca, and arranged for her to come up.

In between all this rushing about Brigie and Kate would spend hours in the sitting room listening to records. I can remember that as early as mid-May, before the exams were over and I was painting the room ready for Jane's twenty-first birthday party, I was having to pick my way with the paint-pots among the lolling figures and their strewn cushions and records. It was very irritating, and Jane remembers that I told her Brigie was testing my patience to the limit. At least, I thought as the summer wore on, her taste in music is quieter than it used to be, with an atmosphere of gentle melancholy that seemed to suit their mood. There was one record that she played repeatedly, for me she said, as I had once expressed an interest in it: Candle in the Wind, about the death of Marilyn Monroe. All the same, I was irked by the lethargy of all this listening, and looked forward to getting our sitting room back into more general use. Once, they were discussing when school would start again after this long break; I reminded Brigie that it would be September 2nd, my birthday, 'And that will be a super present for me,' I said tartly. That turned out to be a bitter irony when I realised that she was suffering not just from lethargy. At that time I wished they would get out and ride the horses for a change. There was Shez up on the Brow, and Brigie seemed to be taking no notice of her. I remember making them go out one day and help with the hay, and felt that at least when Rebecca came there would be more incentive to do some riding.

Her parents, Roger and Marion, brought her in August, at the end of their holiday in Northumberland. It was a very hot day and Brigie was working at the gift shop. We had lunch in the garden, but Rebecca was feeling frail after the massive Tudor meal they had eaten the night before. My hopes for more riding while she was here were unfulfilled: Shez had been shod, becoming lame afterwards, and the sole horse activity was leading her from one small village croft to another as she could not walk on the stony track to the Brow. We had to send for the vet at last, and Shez recovered, but only after Rebecca had gone back.

I learned afterwards that Brigie had told Rebecca that she was worried about being breathless when she went up to the Brow to catch Shez, and even when she went upstairs. She confided that she had even given up smoking. It was only after Brigie started working full-time again at the shop during the last two weeks of August that she mentioned her cough and breathlessness to me. Mary Ann, her great friend there, had become concerned and bought her some cough mixture. I have to admit that I did not take very much notice; everyone had summer colds that year and the coughs seemed to linger on for ages. When Brigie said her side was sore, I thought she had twisted a muscle with the hay-bales. All the same, I intended to make a doctor's appointment for her. G. and I were having a weekend off at Goathland: Jane would look after the post office on Saturday and Brigie on Monday. In the hurry of getting ourselves packed on Friday and the post-office accounts complete, I forgot to ring the surgery. I remembered as we were driving towards the moors, but when we got back on Monday evening Brigie said she felt better and did not need to see the doctor. I accepted this for a couple of days, and then thought that in fact it would be a good idea if she had a check before school started the following week. Brigie said she would go either before work at the shop or late afternoon when she had finished. I was shopping in Skipton that Friday and hoped I could fix an appointment so that I could go with her, but this was not possible. I took Brigie into Skipton, did my shopping, and came home, leaving her to see the doctor before she caught the bus at night.

G. set off to meet her at Lane End in the evening and then the phone rang. It was Mary Ann saying that in view of what the doctor had said Brigie should not think about working the following day. She thought Brigie would already be home and I would know about it. I heard the story from her. Brigie had gone back to the shop after leaving the doctor and she was very upset: he thought her lung might have collapsed. I went cold with shock and guilt; I should have been with her and I should have taken more notice earlier of that cough. Mary Ann had been worried about it before I was, but even she said that she could not believe anything was seriously wrong as Brigie had been working with energy and liveliness during the last two weeks.

Brigie had recovered her calm when she got home. She was to have an X-ray the following morning and go back to the surgery with the plates. Dr. K., our regular doctor, would not be there, but she had an appointment with a senior partner in the practice. Could Kate come with us? she asked.

I realised that Kate's perky presence would be reassuring for her and it certainly helped during the wait for X-rays the next morning. It is unnerving for an adult to sit about those silent, official places worrying about the outcome; how much more for a sixteen year old who had always been very squeamish about illness and physical unpleasantness. We drove off with the plates and waited again at the surgery. Kate had the right comments about things totally un-connected with the situation, and their giggles and jokes together relieved the tension. It became suddenly necessary to swap skirts for some reason, and they rushed into the loos to effect the change with more giggles and larking about. Then Brigie and I were called in. The doctor held up the plates. They showed that Brigie's right lung was two-thirds full of fluid, and in his careful, precise way he said that this was 'important'. I was grateful for his thoughtfulness in not using the word 'serious'. He asked if anyone else in the family had ever had lung problems and I told him about Michael's lobar pneumonia when he was small. This could be something of a similar nature, he thought, but Brigie would have to go to hospital to have it investigated and drained, but not immediately as nothing would happen at the hospital over the Bank Holiday weekend. We went out again to join Kate while he made the arrangements. The thought of hospital was bad enough, but if it meant missing Kilnsey Show on Tuesday that would be disaster for Brigie. She held her breath when he called us back, and huge was the relief when he said she would go on Wednesday, September 2nd, the day school would be starting. I thought of my earlier caustic remark about that day and regretted it.

We came away and went to see Mary Ann; she said again how incredible she found it when she thought of how hard Brigie had worked in the shop. Surely nothing could be badly wrong when she looked and seemed so well. The doctor had also said that she looked very healthy (and Dr. K. told me later that he could not believe that anyone as bouncy as she was could have such a poorly functioning lung) and I tried to believe that this was a temporary alarm which would soon be relieved. It was a good chance, we thought, while we were in Skipton to get some material for Brigie's new school skirt which she was going to make. In the basement at Hartley's Fabrics there was quite a gathering of her school friends to see Claire at her Saturday job. To all of them she announced that she was going to hospital 'to have me lung drained out', the casual and vernacular speech suddenly appearing for her friends. Claire advised the Co-op for material and we found some there, and bought a pattern.

Back in Litton, Val and Dennis suggested taking Kate and

Brigie to Malham Show. It was a welcome relief for them after the morning and Brigie loved seeing the horses. It turned into a lengthy outing as they went on afterwards to have a meal in Settle where Val was introduced to David and Martin. We had both heard about these lads from the girls many times: Brigie and Kate were always on the look-out for a lift to Stainforth's Craven Heifer so that they could see them. The infatuation had begun, I think, at Horton Show earlier in the year, when Brigie and Kate were in the Littondale team for the 'It's a Knock-Out' contest. This involved many hazardous and messy exploits like holding a tray of glasses and walking across a suspended pole greased with Fairy Liquid, trying to avoid the pillows thrown by the other side. The show had satisfied everyone's instinct for enjoying other people's discomfiture and the heavy rain added its contribution as well. They all dried off in the pub afterwards, wet and exhausted. Brigie talked about David for weeks, but I saw him only briefly one afternoon when I collected her and Kate from a fairly entwined group outside the Craven Heifer.

Now he was the main reason for not missing Kilnsey Show. She had not seen him for a week or two (constant diary reference to 'David didn't phone. Very depressed again'). 'If I get on well with him at Kilnsey, Mum, I want him to come and see me in hospital. Would you mind?' This was the only comment she made on next week's programme: indeed when I tried to introduce some reassuring discussion of it that weekend, she said she did not want to talk about it. 'I'm just forgetting about it, until I have to go.' Bank Holiday Monday was quiet and she got on with cutting out her skirt and pinning it together. She got as far as sewing the darts, and putting the zip in place, hoping that it would not be long before she was wearing it. However, I found it impossible to forget about what was pending, and every time that weekend when I looked at her prettiness and her shapeliness there was a feeling of dread. Lung cancer was my unspoken fear. Is this child doomed? I remember asking myself. On reflection, though, it all seemed too melodramatic and too ridiculous and when Ruth Robinson, my friend from Arncliffe, obviously assuming that Brigie might have T.B., told me about her experience of the illness at the same age, I told myself that my thoughts were getting out of hand and I was being silly. Even so, there was always the feeling that if one expected the worst, that in itself was some insurance that it would not happen.

Kilnsey Show day, September 1st, was fine and Brigie was going down with Val, Dennis and Kate. She dressed very carefully in her dark skirt and broderie-anglaise blouse and rejected the idea of a jacket as it would hide the glamour. G. went later to take pictures. The day remained overcast and a very cool wind got up. I was very worried about Brigie being down there in such light clothes and got someone to take a jacket in case they saw her. It seemed to me a very long afternoon: all I wanted now was to get her to hospital so that everything could be put right. She came home eventually, highly elated; she had not been a bit cold, so she said, and she had obviously had a great day with David. Kate came back with her to stay the night and to go with us to hospital in the morning. She had lent Brigie her prettiest nightie and we packed a bag. It was good that she had Kate's company that night. In the morning, she gave me my birthday present, which was from Andrew and Michael as well: a pair of sheepskin gloves which she had chosen some time before to go with the jacket that G. had given me. We set off, leaving him to look after the post office. Jane and Stephen were going to Northumberland for a week.

# 3

○

## Two million to one

Kate's perky comments and giggles kept Brigie going as we
drove along and then made our way to Ward Three. Brigie
was shown a bed and got undressed. There was nobody
about, and in spite of the modern surroundings it was bleak
and cheerless. The other beds in the group of four were
empty, the ladies being in the day room, and Brigie was not
tempted to go in there. She had seen it as we came along—a
group of sick and elderly people sitting silently in their
hospital chairs. A young doctor came to see her while Kate
and I went down to register her, and then she talked to me in
the day room. They suspected T.B., I was told: it was certainly
the most likely explanation of the fluid, and not uncommon
among girls this age. If she had been old they would have
thought of lung cancer, but that would not be the case at her
age. I was startled at the use of this word. Why mention it
merely to discount it? To prepare one for something worse,
or to deal openly with a widespread secret fear? They would
drain her lung and test the fluid. I went back to Brigie and
Kate, and found that the doctor had made the same comment
to Brigie about lung cancer, and thought this was rather
strange.

We had to leave her then, sitting rather helplessly on her
bed wondering what on earth she was going to do all day 'in
this place'. I wondered too; she had some books with her, but

it would not be easy to concentrate in such a strange and unnatural atmosphere. G. and I would come at 7 p.m. We stopped in Skipton and saw Mary Ann briefly and posted a card to reach Brigie in the morning.

Back in Litton, I found Ruth had left a fruit cake for us and a card and bookmark for Brigie ('for all that lovely reading you're going to do in hospital'). She was right in understanding that I would feel very limp, wondering how Brigie was faring in the intervening hours, and suddenly very tired after the tension of the morning. Soon afterwards, Margaret Dagett and Helen came with flowers for Brigie. They knew she was going to hospital, but not exactly when, but Helen had wanted to come to Litton before her school started the next day. Their company was just right for me, quiet and sympathetic as we sat in the garden with Ruth's cake, and then we had a walk round the village for Helen to see all the places that Brigie had talked about. Before they went, Margaret reminded me how important it was to be punctual at the hospital. She had been in hospital and knew how desperately one looked for visitors.

When G. and I got there that night we found Brigie in a state of high excitement. She had been put in a room by herself with her own television, washbasin and loo. 'They think I've got T.B.'—and we might all have to wear gowns and masks when we came to see her. (This 'barrier' nursing, we were told later, would be necessary if it was found that she had the infectious variety of T.B.) G.M. had sent a large bunch of flowers, and with Margaret's as well, the room looked bright and Brigie felt quite important. Two girls from school were there, as they lived just round the corner from the hospital, and they were able to tell her what had happened on the first day back. She liked her little room and television, and we were to bring a *Radio Times*; the nurses were super, young and jolly. All the same, she worried about the draining of her lung which would happen the next day, and after the girls had gone G. sat down and embarked on a long and funny description of all his historic ailments, mostly fairly ludicrous, and Brigie was in fits of laughter at the frequent description of something as 'excruciatingly painful'. G.M. rang her after we had to go, and he did this every night while she was in hospital. She could make calls too, on the portable trolley, and G. left her some coins so that she could ring us when she felt like a chat. I was relieved that night, knowing that she had settled down and had some good company.

I think I rang her the next morning, and she was still cheerful. We were going again in the evening. Dr. Y. had done the first aspiration and she found it quite tolerable. He drew off a litre of fluid through a needle inserted in her back: it gave her only a slight tickle, she said. The fluid looked 'like lager'. After that she went up for an X-ray in a wheelchair. 'I felt a right burk,' she said, and the nurses warned her about the blandishments of the young porter, known as 'Casanova' round the hospital. I was staggered to hear that the X-ray had shown little decrease in the amount of fluid in her lung. Dr. Y. assured me, though, that this was quite under-standable: he was very confident about the ease of treating T.B. She would just take some pills for about ten months, and would probably be well enough to go back to school in a few weeks.

When it came to aspirations with the young doctor things were not so easy. It was accomplished the first time, but it hurt, as there had not been a long enough interval for the freezing to take effect, but the second time the doctor had difficulty finding the right place, which upset Brigie a lot. One knows that young doctors have to learn, but for a sixteen-year-old patient to witness their uncertainty and hear their comments seemed to me inexcusable. Brigie pleaded with me not to say anything about it: she was desperately anxious that I should not 'make a fuss' about any of her discomforts. Making complaints was against my instincts too: the doctor was very pleasant and otherwise very kind to Brigie, but I decided that I had to ensure that Dr. Y. would do all future aspirations. I rang the staff nurse in the morning, as usual, to find out how Brigie was, and he received my comments sympathetically. I was able to tell her that I had been told Dr. Y. would operate in future, without causing her too much worry.

That weekend, Brigie had many visitors. From her window she could see the cars coming down the drive, and we always waved as we arrived, even though we could not see her, and again as we went back home again. Andrew and his friend Mark went on Saturday afternoon, and after the bell rang went round to the outside and talked to her through the window. Instead of being cross with them, someone in authority let Brigie get dressed and go outside and sit on the bank with them. It was very hot weather that September, and often Brigie's little room felt quite stifling. On Sunday afternoon Joanne went with her mother Pat, and Val and Kate. G. and I always went in the evening. Masses of cards had been arriving for her every morning, and her room was full of flowers. She was enjoying all this attention, and looked very pretty lying on her bed in Kate's nightie and her hair curling over her shoulders. The young nurses were great company for her, with their jokes and even wrestling matches in the morning when they insisted that *she* shouldn't be allowed to sleep, when *they* had to work. One of them had a horse and a baby, and we had to take photographs of Shez in to show her. All the same, she was longing to get home again, and we were all longing for a positive diagnosis.

So far, this had not come, in spite of all the tests. I was still worried about cancer, and one night when G. and I went with Michael, we happened to see the sister before we came away. I did not want to be too explicit about my fears in front of Michael, but she assured us very definitely that the chances of Brigie's illness being anything sinister were about two million to one, so remote that they did not even consider it. At the back of my mind there was still the possibility all the same, but it sounded reassuring. They decided to do a bronchoscopy (inserting a tube through her mouth to her lung in order to collect a tissue specimen). It was going to be a big ordeal for her: they did it early one morning and her young nurse friends told her she managed marvellously and boosted her morale. Jane and Stephen came back from Northumberland, and the sister let me take Jane to see Brigie during the day. Jane wrote about it afterwards:

I encountered both Brigie and my mother in a very new, different situation. Brigie, surrounded by flowers, cards, presents, sat like a queen on her bed, her skin slightly jaundiced, and with an unnatural flush to her cheeks, but looking so beautiful I was taken aback. The novelty of so much attention had not worn away and although she had suffered a great deal of pain, she was undoubtedly, as always, on top. She had struck up a great rapport with nurses and doctors; it seemed she was the most important person in the ward, and I felt important to be visiting her. But also, she was now a sick person. She had not looked sick at home. Now surrounded by white walls and bed linen and other sick people, the illness seemed to have gained strength. She talked about the staff and the patients, knew all the medical terms and jargon, a completely new world for her which she had slipped into with apparent ease.

That same evening, Wednesday I think, I saw Dr. Y. after the visiting hour. He said that although they still had no positive results from the tests, they were convinced it was T.B. and would start treatment. Sometimes it was hard to get a positive diagnosis. She would take pills for about nine months, and they would keep a close watch on her through the clinics. She would go back to school in about a month. She could come home at the weekend, probably Saturday. There was just one cold moment for me, when he said something about having to do more tests 'for other things' if this did not work. He dismissed the thought, however, although not quite as de-cisively as the sister had done. Jane and Stephen went to see her on Thursday night, picking up another school friend, Abigail, in Skipton on the way.

On Friday morning Brigie rang me in great excitement: she could come home. I promised I would get down as soon as I could: I think I was as excited as she was as we made our preparations. Brigie's favourite meals had been discussed often during hospital visiting and she had ordered one of G.'s specialities: topside done with button mushrooms and glazed shallots. G. started raiding the freezer as I set off. It was going to be a great celebratory weekend with G.M. and Marilyn coming on Sunday, and G. was intent on doing justice to the occasion.

At the hospital she got into her clothes again and had a final T.B. mantoux test before she left. We were to watch this very closely over the next day or two and let them know how her arm reacted. She felt very shaky and looked very pale, but insisted on stopping in Skipton. One of her friends in the gift shop made a comment which was not entirely helpful. 'Oh, how are you?' she asked. 'You look awful!' She briefly saw one or two of her friends during their lunch-hour from school, and then we came home. The mantoux test was already showing positive. It was lovely to unpack her bag for her and get her established in her own room again after ten days in hospital. The settee in the sitting room was made ready for her to lie on when she got tired, and all her cards were unpacked and the flowers from hospital rearranged. I think she spent some time upstairs watching television in the boys' room that evening. On Saturday morning G. announced that he and Brigie were going to Settle. I was surprised, but I learned later that she had privately asked him to take her. She wanted to buy me a present, she said, 'for being so good to me while I was ill'. He was touched by her bearing in the shop. She had the money she had earned in the gift shop, and was not bothered about the price. She carefully chose the right blouse, and gave me the parcel in the afternoon. Her presentation of it was typically undemonstrative: it was simply 'Here you are, Mum,' but I understood the meaning of it. It was lovely, I said, and the thought behind it even more so. It remains one of my most treasured possessions.

Brigie was still not feeling well, but she went to see Eileen and sat in the kitchen there as she had done so many times before. Eileen remembers that she suddenly went very pale and said, 'I've got to go home now,' and quickly left. Jane offered to go up to the Brow and fetch Shez down for her to see. We watched from the kitchen through the glasses and Brigie laughed as Shez played about and refused to be caught. Jane persisted, though, and they came down the hill in unison. It was great for Brigie to see Shez again, and she led her about and then said she would take her back to the Brow on her own. We had to let her do this, although I was worried that she would not be strong enough to manage her. We were both worried, Jane and I, as she did not come back for ages, but when she came back safely she and Jane went down to the farm. It was a wood-chopping day with the old tree which had fallen some time before quite near Shez's loose-box. Jane was using her camera as they sat on the tractor and watched the operation, and we have pictures of the workers—notably Stewart—hacking and heaving at the heavy wood. Brigie saw Tibby, the new pup, before they came back.

She began to have trouble taking her T.B. pills. They had made her sick once at the hospital, and this difficulty returned. The four-hourly dose became an ordeal, something she had to steel herself for, and the effort of swallowing them seemed to make her sick. She went to bed that night comfortable enough, but after I had been asleep some time I was aware of movement, and found Brigie limping along the passage, crying with a pain in her leg. I knew it must be very severe, because Brigie did not cry easily, and I became very alarmed. I did not know whether aspirin would be compatible with her other drugs, and when the pain continued to be very bad I rang the hospital ward at midnight to ask for advice. It seemed a desperate measure, but I had to get some relief for her, and it was good to hear a steady and non-censorious voice at the end of the line, suggesting that I give her Panadol, and if there was still a problem in the morning to get in touch with our G.P. Fortunately we had some, and that allowed Brigie to get back to sleep. But the problem remained: she was sick again in the morning, and the leg pain was still there. I rang the surgery and spoke to the Sunday duty doctor, and he said to take her in. It was a very distressing journey for her, as the car movement made her feel even more sick. She travelled on the back seat to rest her leg, and hold the basin for her sickness. G. in the meantime was cooking her special meal, though with little heart as it seemed unlikely that she would be able to eat anything.

He in turn had become very alarmed, although he voiced his fears only to me. This new pain in her leg and back reminded him all too vividly of Joan's symptoms. His first wife had been treated for back pain for a long time before they realised she had cancer, and I remembered various people I had known who had one symptom and then another, pains occurring in different parts of the body, inexplicably, until the final dread diagnosis.

Brigie and I went in to see the doctor. He worked very slowly and deliberately, and I could see that Brigie was in great discomfort, and feeling sick again. He said she was feeling transferred pain from pressure on her sciatic nerve and she should go again the next morning for an X-ray on her back. I had my own worries about what might be pressing on her nerve, but could not voice them in front of her. He gave her tablets which he said would help to stop the sickness. By now she was losing all her T.B. tablets, and as the treatment was supposed to be continuous this was very worrying. She had an uncomfortable journey back again, and lay on the settee exhausted with the effort. She stoically took the new pills, with little effect though, and she was very unwell. G.M. and Marilyn had arrived while we were out, but it was a subdued and preoccupied gathering.

The weather was hot and we had our lunch half in the garden and half in the sitting room with Brigie. She was very glad to see them but too uncomfortable to enjoy anything. Marilyn remarked that at least we had this positive mantoux test: that must mean that she had T.B. I was privately unconvinced by this, remembering the tests at school which were to show up the presence, I thought, of a natural T.B. immunity, but which did not necessarily indicate active disease.

The next day she had to face yet another distressing journey with the basin. I drove very carefully, hoping not to give her any jolts, while she was still being sick in the back. My only consolation was that I knew G. was by now ringing Dr. K. to put squarely to him the worry that we felt with this new development. G. had thought out this plan during the night: he would ring while we were on our way, so that by the time Brigie and I got to the surgery with the X-ray plates Dr. K. would know how we felt. It was not something I could explain with Brigie there, and G. would tell him that we had previous experience of cancer not being diagnosed in time, and try to indicate that we were not simply giving way to fanciful and emotional anxieties.

Brigie struggled up the stairs and down again, and with the plates we went back to the surgery. We carried the basin everywhere: the nurse let her lie down in her room and Dr. K. came to see her there. He and his colleague looked at the plates together, but they found nothing worrying. There was just a possibility that one slightly misshapen vertebra was causing the trouble, but they thought it unlikely. Dr. K. looked at me very intently and said firmly he could find no cause for anxiety 'at all, at all, at all'. By this emphasis I knew he was responding to G.'s telephone call. Pains like this often resulted from a spell in hospital, change of bed, simply feeling poorly. I should rub her back with Transvasin. She should persist with the T.B. pills and the sickness would very likely go. Again, it seemed reassuring. G. had found him sympathetic and understanding about our worries, and he was at pains to allay them.

But the sickness and the pains did not go. I slept in Brigie's room and rubbed her back and leg as the pain woke her during the night. It made no difference. I took G. to the train early on Tuesday morning and went back to the surgery, hoping to catch Dr. K. before he started work. He told me he would ring the hospital and ask advice about the continuing sickness. Brigie was still in bed when I got back, and was very upset at the prospect of having to go back to hospital. I felt absolutely wretched about it too, and yet I knew she could not go on like this. When the surgery rang, later that morning, to say that she should go back the following day I was the one who cried when I went upstairs to tell her. My lapse possibly did her good: she had to comfort me. 'Oh, don't cry, Mum. It'll be all right,' and she held up her arms to hug and reassure *me*. I remember that I was telling Janet Beard later when she came in, and I cried again, the only time in the shop, I think. Val and Brenda came in during the morning and offered to look after the post office for half the morning each while I went with Brigie. Jane had gone to Edinburgh to stay with Helen for a few days.

Brigie slept in my bed that night, and as the pain increased I would try to ease it with the liniment. I knew it was having no effect but it was better for both of us to feel that something was being done. I think we were not bothering with the T.B. pills: there seemed no point when they just made her sick. We got ready in good time and drearily repacked her bag. I asked her whether she wanted me to put in all her 'get well' cards again: she said no, and indeed they seemed out of date by this time. I was feeling hopeful again, though; surely they would try some new pills that would not upset her system and then she would be home again before long and for good. She sat in the kitchen ready to go that morning, and Andrew was there too: feeling her depression, I was saying that she would just be in for a day or two, until they got her treatment sorted out. She indicated that she did not want any more discussion: she got up and said quietly, 'Right, then,' and we went out to the car.

She was in Ward Three again, but not in the little room. In

fact, she was next to an old lady whose constant sickness had revolted her the previous week. I felt very depressed with this arrangement, but in fact it was good: this was Mrs. Johnson from Stainforth, and Brigie discovered that she knew David and Martin and they got on very well. She liked having company. I had collected the back and leg X-rays from the surgery and taken them with us, and I was worried that the staff seemed uninterested in these pains, but relieved when she was put on new T.B. drugs and she stopped being sick. They told her that as soon as she went twenty-four hours without sickness she could come home again, and she was determined to achieve this goal. This was a battle that she won, and by Friday I was collecting her again. I think we stopped at Ruth's on the way back and Brigie saw her splendid doll's house.

So she came home again, for good as we thought. In ten days' time, on September 28th, she would go for a check at the clinic, but in the meantime various events were planned and she wanted to finish her school skirt. Derek's party was that night, but Brigie did not feel up to that, and she and Kate watched television together. It was a quiet and relaxed time and we looked forward to Brigie's improvement continuing. She was still limping with the pain in her leg, but not so badly, and the T.B. pills were being tolerated. It was good for her to catch up with people and happenings in Litton, and to be able to join in what was going on. It must have been a horrid feeling for her to know that life was going on without her all that time. That was how it seemed to all of us, I think: in terms of emotion and strain a very long time, but by the calendar just three weeks since she went to the doctor for that first, fairly casual check.

Mark and Andrew had promised to take her to Lister's when she came out of hospital, a celebratory dinner to start her return to normal life. It was, however, a watershed time for several others as well: Andrew was soon to begin his course at Bangor University, Jane was going back to Goldsmith's, and Derek, another friend, was leaving soon for a year's work in New Zealand and Canada. Quite a party set off for Malham on Tuesday night—with Jean and John from Pen-y-Ghent and Stewart and his wife Sandra joining in along with Mark, Stephen and Kate. They all had a great evening: the staff constructed one large table for them at the end of the room and they themselves joined in the hilarity. Brigie loved it.

Various other quietly pleasurable things happened that week. On Wednesday I had to go shopping in Keighley and Jane and Brigie came too. We went to Marks and Spencer's first, and I remember thinking at the time how lovely it was to be out with my two daughters again; it was a long time since we had all been on an expedition together. We bought tea towels for Andrew to take to Bangor, and we chose pants for the girls ('I really love getting new pants,' Brigie said) and then we met one of Brigie's nurse friends out with her baby. I had to go to the cash-and-carry and Brigie came in with me, 'to keep an eye on you', as she put it, as I was apt to get carried away and buy too many 'new lines' for the shop. I noticed that she was still breathless as she insisted on collecting my boxes of goods, holding her mouth closed in concentration to economise on the breath in her nostrils. She had enough energy, though, to protest as I hovered over a box of canned red cherries. 'You'll never sell those, Mum!' She clicked her tongue and threw up her eyes in mock desperation as I put them on the trolley. 'Do you know what she collected today?' she told Jane back in the car. 'She does need watching. I had to drag her away.' I think of those remarks every time I see the cherries still sitting on the shelf.

Thursday, the day before Kate's sister's wedding: Jane went down to Amerdale House to help Val with the flowers, and Andrew looked after the post office while Brigie and I went to Settle to collect Sarah's wedding cake. We had to bump past the road-widening machines on Barks as we went over and I wondered how we would get the cake back without damage. However, the baker got it firmly established on the back seat and Brigie guarded it during the journey home. The next morning Sarah rang to ask her to go to the wedding itself and she was delighted. It was another beautiful day for the ceremony, the last, as it turned out, of that warm and golden autumn. Val remembers that she was still limping as they went out to have photographs taken, and when I joined them in the evening at East Garth I thought she looked very pale. It would be a relief to get her to the clinic on Monday, as it seemed these new pills were not doing their work.

Brigie's breathlessness was even more obvious the next day, Saturday. Stephen was taking Jane back to London and Andrew was going, too, to stay with G.M. for a day or two. He and Michael were beating in the morning, but the weather had broken and the rain was pouring down. The shoot was called off and they would have left early if it had not been for the floods. By early afternoon the dub had 'come out'. This is the local description of the gush of water that pours from the slope below the farm after very heavy rain and leaves eighteen inches of water standing on the road. It takes a certain expertise and nerve to get through it by car. There was a long debate in our kitchen about the possibility of floods lower down the dale, and Stephen decided to risk it. As they set off into all that wetness Brigie and I went out to see Shez. She was in the small croft across the road, and was shivering with cold and wet, and Brigie said she must have a bran mash. We went down to the farm to collect the ingredients and passed Kate's horse Sultan, cold and wet in his field. As we came up the road Brigie had to ask me not to go so fast: she was out of breath and her leg was sore. Brigie was tired as Shez gratefully wolfed her meal, but she insisted that we must give Sultan a mash as well, as Kate was still at work. I was very conscious of the determined and deliberate way she was going about these tasks and could see that it was a great effort for her. It was while we were coming up the slope from the farm for the second time, with Brigie really struggling, that she noticed Stephen's car return to the other side of the dub and a familiar figure—Jane—get out and start scrambling for the wall to take the high muddy way across the field. She came in a few minutes later, dripping and saturated: true to her nature, inherited from me, she had forgotten some vital materials for college. We had a good laugh at her as she set off for the second time through the torrents and the mud.

# 4

## Summer's end

It really felt now like the end of the summer: the rain seemed to have washed out the quiet autumnal mellowness. Jane had gone back. Andrew would go in a week, and Brigie would go to the clinic on Monday. I knew the treatment was not working, but concentrated on the doctor's previous comment that sometimes T.B. drugs took some time to reduce the fluid on the lung. As Dr. Y. discovered from her X-ray that Monday afternoon her lung was still full: she would have to go back into hospital. Brigie's first reaction was not as depressed as I feared it would be: I think we both knew inwardly that a return would be required and we were braced. Much as she wanted to be at home she got very depressed when she was too unwell to do all the home things: that was nearly as isolating as actually being cut off in hospital. A phone call later in the day said that she should go in the morning to Ward One. When Kate came up as usual to see her after work she said she would try to get the day off so that she could come too. This turned out to be impossible, but in fact Brigie was by now fairly experienced at going into hospital and had progressed beyond the stage of needing bright and lively conversation to take her mind off the unpleasantness. It was a different atmosphere from the first time: now I felt there was a resignation that she had to face the reality of being ill.

As we waited in the kitchen the next morning with the yet

again repacked bag, Andrew came through on his way to the farm, the sort of departure that Brigie had made so many times before. He was going off fairly casually, and as he went through the door Brigie called out, 'Have a nice time at college,' and she was crying. It was useless for me to say that he would see her before he left: the incident epitomised everything that she was feeling. Everyone else was going out into the world, but she was going back to hospital, yet again. G. too was going to London, and we left him at the station on the way to Airedale. I felt her depression beside me as we went along. I wanted to put her in touch with a deeper support that I knew, but which we had not talked about before. I told her that I would be with her as much as I could, and that even in absence I would be thinking about her all the time. And then I told her that prayer was very important to me, that I would be praying for her and many other people were doing so, and I believed very strongly that it would help her. She did not comment, and I did not say more.

Her spirits were still very low when we got to Airedale and went through the familiar routine of registration and making our way to the ward. She was put out in the ward with old ladies again. I think it was then that I asked if I could come in the afternoons and they agreed when I explained that this was her third time of coming to hospital and she was depressed. It seemed better for me to go then, and other visitors at night—the afternoons were long and empty as the old ladies went to the day room which she hated. By the second day, she said she preferred the ward to the single room as there was more to see and people to talk to. The young doctor often came and sat on her bed and told her the news from Ward Three. The nurses there were sorry that Brigie had not gone back to them: Mrs. Johnson had been moved upstairs and had had her leg amputated. This was not very cheering news, but Brigie liked the contact with the friendly doctor. She gradually got to know the old ladies: there was one diagonally across who was very dogmatic and irritating, but Clara, next to her, caught her sympathy. She had been asleep when we first arrived, surrounded by high cot barriers to prevent her falling. Brigie told me, one afternoon, that Clara had been crying quite a lot. Brigie confessed that she didn't know what to do when Clara cried, but she'd given her a tissue and then a sweet. I said I thought that was just right. Brigie herself cried sometimes during these days when we were alone. I would draw my chair close up to her and we would 'go into a huddle' as we called it, so that no one else would see her tears. She could cry only with me, she said: no one else should see her out of control. In the evening she would be bright and chirpy with whoever came: a rota of visitors was arranged by telephone. 'Mark will come,' said Brigie. 'I know he will—and Abigail,' and we knew that Kate would be as staunch as ever.

Brigie was still getting a lot of pain in her leg and was not sleeping well. The staff did not seem to take the pain seriously, but she got very cross and distressed when I tried to talk to them about it. She was still very anxious that I should not 'make a fuss' and I ended by voicing my anxieties to them on the telephone in the morning when I rang. I knew that Brigie was being very stoical about her discomfort: she was not a plaintive teenager, and was making little to them of the pain which she undoubtedly felt. All this time Dr. Y. was giving her more aspirations, and they were trying to find out why the fluid was still accumulating. There was to be a case conference about Brigie, he said, in which all the specialists would be consulted. G. went to see her on his own on Thursday evening and talked afterwards to the staff nurse: he found him very nervous and evasive, although he did not tell me at the time.

On Friday, I went in the afternoon, intending to stay, and found Brigie dressed and ready to come home for the weekend. Although that was a very good prospect for her she was taking time. She was sitting on the edge of Clara's bed: it was a beautiful scene in which I saw a new Brigie. Clara was lying there, and they were just looking at each other. I tried to join in the slow conversation that was going on, but soon realised that my remarks were clumsy and useless. Brigie was in touch with the slow rhythm and the need of this old lady: she was not saying much, just smiling and responding as needed.

'I don't like being here,' Clara said.

Brigie considered this for some time. 'I think you do like it really—it's better than being on your own.'

'But I don't like it without you,' and the sad old eyes became even more watery.

'But I'll be back on Monday—it isn't very long at all.'

There was another long pause.

'We look after each other,' Clara said.

'We prop each other up,' said Brigie.

Another pause. Clara looked up at me, and then back at Brigie. 'You've got a good mother,' she said.

Then the old, mocking Brigie came to the fore. 'You should see her sometimes when she's telling me off,' she said with a laugh.

Here the irritating old lady opposite joined in, breaking the sensitivity. 'You shouldn't talk like that about your mother, Brigid. I'm sure she's very good to you.'

After that we could only say goodbye to Clara, and Brigie promised to see her on Monday morning. It was a contrast with the last time I had collected her from hospital. Then another old lady had pinned me with a long and rambling tale of her miseries and Brigie was very embarrassed when I nearly cried for her. 'She says that to everyone, Mum, and it's not true. You shouldn't take any notice of her.' Brigie, it seemed, had developed a new and sensitive insight into old ladies, and showed me the ineptness of my bumbling efforts.

She did not feel like stopping in Skipton this time, and when we got back to Litton she sat in the kitchen feeling very unwell, even wondering if it had been a good idea to come home at all. I got the settee ready for her and she spent most of the weekend there. G.M. was coming on Sunday, in order to drive Andrew to Bangor, and that was something for Brigie to look forward to. He slept in Brigie's room, on Jane's bed, that night and was very worried that she was still getting so much pain in her neck and leg. He would take Brigie to Airedale in the morning on the way to Bangor. He wrote to her again when he got back to Broxbourne, and after describing Andrew's room in Bangor he went on:

It was smashing to see you again, though I hope to see you before long without hospital hovering in the background. Mum says that they're giving you more powerful painkillers to help you sleep better, which is *good*. You're a very brave, super girl (as well as a lot of other special things) and I'm very proud to be your father. Without maybe realising it you're doing something that very few people ever manage to do; which is to set a tremendous example to the rest of us in how to cope with a difficult, rather scary and unpleasant situation. I mean that, Brigie. Not one of us in this strange rambling interconnected family of ours will ever, if ill, be able to avoid trying to measure up to you. If Brigie could be cheerful and strong, we shall say to ourselves, when *she* was feeling rotten, then we *must*. It's very rare for anyone to have that sort of effect on other people, but you do and will. Salute!

Don't get too worried about all the prodding and poking that doctors may do. Unpleasant while it's happening, but reassuring to know that it will get to the bottom of the trouble and presently put it right. The only thing I'm worried about is how much leeway you're going to have to make up when you get back to school—and how ropable Shez might be after several weeks without you on her back. Will you, incidentally, start thinking what etc for Xmas, birthday and all that? They'll be putting the decorations up in Regent Street before we know where we are, heaven help us.

I went to see her in the afternoon, and arranged to see Dr. Y. that evening at the beginning of the visiting hour. Kate was coming with me and she talked to Brigie while I saw the doctor. He said he was still convinced she was suffering from T.B. but as she was not responding to treatment they would have to test for 'other things'. I asked if that meant malignancy and he said yes. There was nothing more he could say at this stage, but I should see him again the following evening after the visiting hour.

I went in to Brigie. Kate was still with her and they were looking at the photos of Sarah's wedding. Kate went off to see Suzanne Aldersley who was in the maternity ward. I remember concentrating very hard on putting aside my own turmoil. Brigie was questioning me very closely about what Dr. Y. had said. She was always very distrustful when any doctor asked to speak to me alone, and I had to be very careful to give her a full and calm account of nearly everything the doctor had said: that they were trying to find out why the T.B. pills were not reducing the fluid in her lung, that they might have to put her on to other pills, that they still believed she had T.B. and that sometimes it took a while for them to get the right treatment sorted out. It was a positive relief that night when the bell went and it was time to go. I think I left Brigie without any additional fears, but I could not be sure. I still had to talk to Kate all the way home, when what I needed most was time to get my own thoughts into some sort of order. It was a relief to talk to G. about it on the phone and later to tell G.M. We still had to cling to the fact that no one had yet said there was evidence of malignancy. I spoke to Helen in Edinburgh too, as I had done many times before: it was useful to talk to those with some medical experience. Marilyn's father had been very helpful as well all this time in giving me a fuller explanation of T.B. and its treatment than I had gleaned from the hospital.

The day after, October 6th, I was picking Kate up again and taking her to the hospital with me. G. was coming home that night, but there would be an hour to wait for him at the station after visiting and I suggested that Kate come home with Colin Aldersley instead. Fortunately she arranged this. We talked to Brigie together and then Kate went up to

Suzanne. It seemed a long hour to me before the bell rang and a nurse came to tell me that Dr. Y. was waiting. I was collecting my things and saying goodbye to Brigie, but she insisted that I leave my bag there so that I could come and see her afterwards. I followed the nurse into the doctor's room and heard her telling him about the bag. He spoke to me very quietly and gently: they had found some 'highly suspicious' cells in the lung fluid and in the pleura, the lung lining, and there was a lesion on her left hip bone. The words were unfamiliar and indirect: was he telling me, I asked, that Brigie had cancer? He said, 'Yes, and we think it's in the bone.' I remember staring very hard at the pattern of the curtains behind him. Ordinary things like the window-frame and the telephone suddenly looked very strange. A different person outside myself was going on asking questions and listening to that quiet voice. They would be doing a great number of tests now to find the primary source: she had already had an internal examination and there was nothing wrong there. The case conference had produced no explanation: they were still puzzled. Even as I asked my last question I knew it was futile. 'What do you think of her chances?'

'I think they are good,' he said, but I knew he had no firm reason for that opinion.

I told him that I had promised to tell her what he had said. He suggested saying that they had found some cells in her body which were multiplying too fast and that she would on Thursday see a specialist in this condition. We would be there too.

Somehow I had to go back to Brigie then. Dr. Y. had obviously tried to spare me that ordeal, but she had thwarted his plans. I was determined not to show her any of the shock I was feeling. I told her about the tests they were going to do and said we would talk about it more the next day. I think that other outside part of me managed to do this without causing alarm to her, and it was only when I got back, mercifully alone, to the safety of the car that I could allow the separate parts of me to come together again. There was still the drive to Skipton to be accomplished, and I took it very deliberately, concentrating very hard on the road and keeping the appalling information at bay until I came to a stop outside the station.

That hour on my own was much needed. I had to get myself in order, and try to control my pounding pulses. Too shattered to cry, I tried to pray and managed a little, but there were terrors when I started to imagine how it might go on. Even so, there came a conviction that we would be helped to cope with this in the right way, even though at that time I felt totally weak and helpless. This hour quietly alone was very important, and about fifteen minutes before G.'s train I was able, reassuringly, to make one minor decision. I would go and ring G.M. from a call-box—that would be easier than doing it at home—and I would buy some alcohol and cigarettes. The latter had helped me over earlier crises, and I would accept help in any way at all. G.M. took the news calmly and quietly and asked me if I thought I would be able to sleep that night. I said I thought I would. It seemed very strange to be doing an ordinary, normal thing like dialling a telephone number, shopping and accepting change, when the world seemed suddenly totally abnormal. Back at the station, hating the taste of my first cigarette for six years (but I'm going to persist with it, I thought) I realised that it was necessary to concentrate on the immediate task, and not to waste nervous energy in allowing the vast and overwhelming tide of future uncertainties to advance into the consciousness: that way one could drown.

G. knew there was something wrong as soon as he saw the cigarette. Though terribly distressed, he, too, took the news calmly and we started for home. I wanted to get back to that safe place as quickly as possible, and again I went very carefully and deliberately. G. wanted to drive, but I knew I was capable of doing it: I had had that hour of quiet. When we got back to Michael I had to become two people again but it was a relief to concentrate on the small events of his still fairly normal life. I remember going into some detail about what he would like for breakfast the next day and about his dinner money. Behind this, too, was the knowledge that Michael was much on his own with all this hospital visiting and me not being here for meals: even though he was going to Eileen or Val or Sandra, he must be feeling left out. And the strain must be obvious to him, but as yet we could not talk about it. Nobody could know until Brigie herself knew. When Michael went to bed G. rang G.M. They would come on Friday or possibly Thursday to see the specialist with us.

The night was very broken: we would sleep for a short time and then the heavy thumping in my chest would wake me. It was a relief to come down and sit quietly in the kitchen, think, and pray for Brigie in her hospital bed and pray for us all, just the short 'Please help us' which was all I was capable of. Nor was I capable of serious thought, but the conviction grew that we would be given strength to take one step at a time and to do our best for Brigie. We must help her to fight this illness: her state of mind and will to live would be very important. G. would join me and make another cup of tea, and then we would try to sleep until the racing pulses set me on the move again. At some stage during the night I thought of the nuns at Fairacres. They and their Mother Mary Clare had supported me through an earlier crisis: I would write to the new Mother-General in the morning.

We could not visit Brigie during the next day as she was having too many tests and a liver biopsy. I found that it was calming to be outside, and I spent as much time as I could that day in the garden, cutting down the old raspberry canes. As I worked plans began to emerge: we would speak to one or two people who would be able to help us, Ruth and Canon Slaughter for a start. He must have experience of guiding people through the problems of serious illness. Most of all, I wanted to talk about how I was to tell Brigie that she had cancer. I remembered past reading: information can be given in response to questions. How would I know the right time and how find the right words? I spoke to Helen in Edinburgh: she was sure, she said, that the words would come naturally. But in the interval, how was I going to hide my strain and the fact that I was keeping information from Brigie even for a short while?

G. and I went to see her at night. The liver biopsy had been very painful indeed. I had not realised what was involved. She was very pleased that everyone was amazed that she had managed so well. 'Cor, it really hurt, you know. I held on to that nurse's hand really hard.' We told her that there seemed to be some areas in her body, like the lung and the hip, where cells were multiplying too quickly and they had to find a cause of this. A specialist would see her the next day and we would be there too. G. privately thought that her own knowledge of biology would point to the implications of this, but she accepted the information seemingly without worry, and was quite bright and cheery when we left.

We went on to Bolton Abbey and talked to Maurice Slaughter in his little room there, stopping for some rather unpalatable fish and chips on the way. He was very kind but I found it difficult to get my thoughts in order and have any kind of rational discussion. I was very glad that G. was there: he and Maurice had some rather academic discussion about being 'agnostic' about Brigie's illness. The thought was too abstract for me then; what I wanted was guidance about how to tell her that she had cancer, but I realised that no one could solve this problem for me. Several suggestions he made that night were very helpful in other ways.

'The parents' attitude of hope,' he said, 'is vital. You have to say to her, in effect, "Look, *live!*" ' and he mentioned a case where the parents had given up hope and the child died. 'Much will depend on you, and she will take her strength from you. You must husband your resources and not waste energy on long conversations with other people. Talk only to those who can help you. Nourish your own selves to replace the energy that you are giving her: listen to music, have time to be quiet, or read a little. You have to be resource-full people, so that you can support her.' About telling Brigie the truth he said, 'Be honest, but don't depress her.' The tightrope still seemed to me very difficult to negotiate. He would come if we needed him day or night, he said. 'If there's chaos, just ring.' I was grateful for his sensitivity. He would be at Airedale the following day, and we should meet him after we had seen the specialist.

G. had wondered whether I should cancel the coffee morning I had arranged on Thursday for Jill and Shirley, two recent arrivals in the village, but I decided to go ahead with it. It was best, I felt, to try to carry on as normally as possible, and it was a distraction for me, nervous as I was about seeing the specialist in the afternoon. We closed the post office that afternoon and found the consulting room at the hospital. Brigie was having an X-ray, we learned, and would come later. We waited in that bare corridor for a very long time, very anxious and nervous, and I remember how good it was that everyone who passed along smiled at us. It was a small matter, but an important and relaxing communication of warmth. Eventually Brigie was pushed along carrying her X-ray plates and wearing her old brown dressing gown. We sat with her in the waiting room and then we all went in to meet a tall, white-coated man with very blue eyes surrounded by many wrinkles. He was pleasant with Brigie. 'Now then, young Brigid,' and he smiled. She lay on the bed with two nurses standing by and he felt all her glands. It was a relief of tension to have a joke about Brigie being ticklish. He asked her if she felt pain, and she mentioned her 'sciatica'. That was all. She was taken back to the ward. We followed him into his office.

It was a difficult interview. All he would say was that they did not know enough yet: they would do a bone biopsy on her hip and analyse the sample. He would see what Brigie's doctor said. This doctor was a stand-in for the consultant who was away during all this period. He did mention casually that her liver seemed to be enlarged, although this could come from the pressure of fluid on her lung. The doctor was clearly interested in the disease, though not anxious to talk about it to the parents. It was just as well that G.M. had not come up as he had thought of doing: Dr. Y. had advised that little would emerge from this consultation and he was right. We met Maurice briefly and told him what had happened. He would be seeing Brigie in hospital, he said. I asked her later whether she liked seeing Canon Slaughter (she had no natural affinity with clergymen). 'Oh yes,' she said. 'I think he's sweet.'

We went back to the ward and found Brigie lying on her bed, looking more lost and lonely than I had ever seen her before. She wanted to know what the doctor had said to us, and we could truthfully say not much. G. left us alone as Brigie felt very low. I pulled my chair up close, and she cried. 'It was just a waste of time,' she said, 'he didn't do anything at all.' We talked about the tests they were going to do. I knew all this waiting was miserable indeed, and she was being so good, I said. When she had recovered from her tears her eyes were searching my face for comfort and meaning, but she did not ask any questions. I stayed there until the hospital tea time and then G. and I went back to Skipton and had a meal at a Chinese restaurant. It was pointless going back to Litton before visiting that evening.

R.A.F. Dave was going as well, I knew, driving a Land-Rover slowly down from Hubberholme where he was having more exercises. It was good that he was there that night: Brigie sparkled away for him and it eased our strain. He told her about the helicopter that was coming to give her a ride. We hoped desperately that this would happen, but we carried that burden of information that no one else knew.

Ruth was coming to see us on Friday morning. G. was looking after the shop and joined in as he could. She had two experiences, she said, that she wanted to share with us because she felt they were relevant. The first was when her daughter, Catherine, was a baby: she was born with a faulty valve in her throat and was unable to digest food. Ruth and John decided against an operation as it was too risky for such

85

a tiny child, and the doctors advised that a diet of Bengers food was then the only thing that would keep her alive. Catherine hated it, and every meal became a struggle with Ruth herself very tense and saying to herself, 'I *will* save my child.' The tension and the struggle went on, but Catherine was not growing. John suggested a service of laying-on of hands. He was ministering at Wells where they lived in the Bishop's Close, and they and the other clergy took Catherine into the small chapel there. During the service Ruth felt the tension ease out of her: she took Catherine home, gave her normal food, and she flourished. The healing had been for her, not the baby, she felt. It was her own intense anxiety and the feeling that everything depended on her that needed the healing. The other experience was when she was in hospital with a cerebral haemorrhage just after John had become Bishop of Woolwich: he had to tell her that she had only a fifty-fifty chance of survival. In spite of the fact that she had four small children, a great calm came over her and she had a very strong feeling that 'whatever happens, all will be well.'

She went on to say that physical death was not a disaster, but a 'cancer of the soul' was. Families often experienced a great closeness during these times. I knew this to be so from my own reading, and had wondered in the past if we as a family would be able to meet the death of one of us in a positive way. I was, however, not prepared to accept this as our experience now: we must concentrate on helping Brigie to live. Her death was unthinkable.

I was calmed by Ruth's wise suggestion that my own inner trust and confidence 'that all would be well' would be transferred to Brigie. This was not, she said, an easy optimism but the much deeper hope: a distinction which John often emphasised. This applied to my conversation with Brigie: if I worried about saying the right thing, or not saying the wrong thing, I would create tension. 'It is better to say the wrong thing out of calm and confidence than the right thing in a tense way. The "wrong" words may produce an opening and a release which you can build on.' She talked about being quiet and empty inwardly, getting rid of the 'clutter' in the mind which leads to confusion and weariness. It linked with Maurice's words about resources.

These two conversations—with Maurice and Ruth—had been very helpful. There were other helpful people too. I spoke to Paul (Brigie's godfather) in Derby, and he suggested getting in touch with Jane Davies whose young daughter had died of cancer. She had become very informed on the treatment of cancer, particularly for the young, and she promised me all help when she knew more about the type that Brigie had. The panic and the tension would still reappear, especially when I thought of what I was going to say to Brigie, but I began that day using the drive to the hospital as a time for conscious quietness, going down into myself, allowing at the best times (it did not always work) a power of love and strength into the vacuum. Already I knew that prayers were being offered and I had a strong sense that we were being held as in a net. When I felt sufficiently calm I would try to concentrate my thoughts on Brigie, to imagine how it felt for her and to try to understand her need, so that when I got to the hospital I would be able to respond to her, rather than be distracted with my own anxieties.

G. had stayed at home this Friday afternoon to do the post-office balance and to cook a meal for us. G.M. and Marilyn were coming to stay the night. Brigie told me about the bone scan which she had found an interesting process. The heavy equipment had passed slowly above her prone form. 'Sister says I'm radioactive now!' The prospect of the bone biopsy on Monday was not comfortable: they were intending to do it with a local anaesthetic and she tried not to think about it. She was still full of these experiences and was not asking any questions, although the doctors too were giving her plenty of opportunity to do so. On Saturday morning she would come home for the weekend.

That Friday evening the four of us had our first opportunity to discuss her illness. Decisions would have to be taken about treatment, and G. decided to get back for the following

Thursday in case we had to see the specialist again. I was profoundly grateful for this, knowing that he would be talking to the doctor with me: I could never remember the right questions to ask, and he always thought clearly and could probe. I had a horror of being swept into agreement to chemotherapy with all its hideous side-effects. This was a feeling shared by all four of us—grave doubts about the standard treatments for a disease which was still so little understood. We remembered Joan's ordeal. It was the first of many alcohol-laced discussions under clouds of cigarette smoke (the alcohol helped to relax us and no one ever had too much) and as the evening wore on there was a feeling of solidarity that was important to all of us. We would find out all we could about alternative treatments. Marilyn could get the books and she and G.M. would digest them: he would talk to a friend who had successfully fought off cancer with a special diet. We would all ask the medical people we knew, Dr. K. himself, a friend in Hoddesdon, and Marilyn's father. It was all fairly abstract, as we did not have a prognosis, but it was a good feeling to have a concerted approach.

I went in for Brigie on Saturday morning. She was still taking the T.B. pills and sleeping pills because of the pain. Her two days were spent on the settee, and we were trying to get her to eat: it was an effort and she still felt sickly. Brigie's main desire was for potato soup ('Zuppa di patata' in my Italian recipe book) and everyone during these several weeks had to consume it, too. There was not time to make separate dishes. Brigie was getting worried about Shez being cold on her hill and Marilyn and I went up to put the New Zealand rug on her. We felt quite pleased with ourselves, even though I did have to come back and ask Brigie's advice about the straps. G. and G.M. stayed with Brigie and Mark and Kate came to see her. On Sunday G.M. and Marilyn went back to Kirkby Overblow to talk to Dr. Edwards and then on to Broxbourne. I had to ring the hospital on Sunday because we had run out of sleeping pills. G. had to go down to Airedale for more and sister said Brigie should not eat or drink after midnight in case they wanted to give her a general anaesthetic for the bone biopsy. This possibility was more reassuring for her. Neil came that day, too, and took her for a drive in his new car.

Her drive the next day did not have the same pleasure: it was back to Airedale yet again. I parked as close to the door as I could, but I should have got a wheelchair for the journey down the long corridor. Brigie had to stop innumerable times to get her breath back, but she was still desperate that I should not make a fuss. She was going for her operation which would be in two parts, I was told: a bone biopsy on her hip and a lung biopsy to see if that revealed anything about the nature of the cancer. I came home and wrote to Jane and Andrew trying to prepare them for bad news. Brigie was still very sleepy from her operation when we got back to the hospital in the evening. Dr. Y. said she could come home again as soon as the effects of the anaesthetic had worn off. It would take them nearly a week to analyse the sample of bone tissue, so she should return to Airedale on the following Monday. It was possible, he suggested, that she would ask me questions when she was at home for this length of time.

I went in for her on Tuesday. We had by now arranged with the Post Office that we could close in the afternoons while Brigie was ill. People like Val and Ruth and Brenda had been very kind in keeping it open, but I knew the village would understand when the need to go to hospital was so urgent, or simply to have more time with Brigie at home. I wondered what other people were making of it all: Steve told us of the concerned conversations at the pub about 'what that girl is going through'.

Some of them, I thought, must suspect that she had cancer, but we had to go on with the cool remarks about 'more tests to find the right drugs' and all the other forms of words that we developed during this period. No one must know before Brigie herself knew. Colin once said, 'Well, she's got that fight in her,' and I wondered if he suspected.

Brigie and I decided that she should sleep on the settee

because the stitches in her hip would be painful on the stairs. I would join her with a mattress on the floor, and once again she had to endure my snoring. I would wake to hear this voice saying, 'Mum, do you think you could stop snoring?' in varying degrees of irritation, and I tried very hard to let her get to sleep again first after I had helped her to the outside loo during the night, so that she would be unaware of my noises. She usually had some wry comments to make in the morning: 'You were going really well last night!' G. vowed *he* did not snore, so perhaps he should stay with Brigie, but we both listened to him sometimes, and his pleasantly distant trumpetings from our room above. My snoring was only one of her discomforts: her stomach was distended with the pressure of the fluid and this made sitting up uncomfortable; she was being sick again with the T.B. pills (how I longed for them to be stopped as their only value was psychological). The weights and measures people came on Wednesday morning to check our scales, and I can remember going in and out with a basin while they were here. She couldn't enjoy even her favourite foods which we were more than ready to make for her, and sometimes after a bout of exhausting sickness she would say, 'It isn't fair, is it?' This was the strongest complaint she ever made, but there were several times during that week when she was overcome by the sheer misery of being ill so long, and I would weep with her as I tried to give her some comfort. Once she cried and said that she 'couldn't even talk to Michael now'; 'I can't even remember what it feels like to be well.' How long, did I think, before she could go back to school? I said she would probably need treatment for this problem of the multiplying cells ('I must be a very active person,' she said) and after that she should be able to go to school. 'Perhaps after half-term?' she asked. I thought that would probably be too soon. She decided she might have to give up biology: it was difficult anyway and it would be hard to catch up now. One beautiful autumn afternoon she looked through the front window and said, 'That hill looks so lovely and all I can do is lie here.' I wanted to say that we would get her up there somehow, but it would not have been kind. I longed to be able to talk to her openly but she was not ready yet.

Perhaps it was the same afternoon that Andrew rang, and by his casual 'thanks for the letter', I knew that he had not taken in its message. He told me quite a lot about the college, how his timetable was working out, and about the other students in the hall. Finally he asked brightly, 'How's every-one?' My letter had certainly failed to communicate. I just said that Brigie was not very well, and doing a bit of quick calculation suggested that he come home for the weekend in ten days' time: by then surely I would be able to tell him and Jane what was wrong.

Jane, on the other hand, was worried by my letter and thought she should come home on Friday. Stephen had planned to go down to her that weekend and I urged him to do so, partly because he needed a break, but mainly because I could not face actually seeing Jane and not telling her the truth. It was one thing to talk evasively and cheerfully on the phone, but face-to-face contact was quite another, and I knew Jane would sense the strain anyway. Michael was having to live with it, but he was out a lot on his own pursuits, going up to the moor with Dennis at the weekends and helping at the farm after school. People told me afterwards that he was very quiet during this period and did not want to answer any of their questions about Brigie. This, I think, was probably the worst period for him.

So things stood on Friday, October 16th. Stephen was going down to see Jane in London. Gladys and Dick, the children's grandparents, were coming in the afternoon to see Brigie. They had been desperately anxious all this time and every day Dick had sent a postcard, usually one from his precious collection of very old cards, collectors' pieces, as he said. His diary entries for this time show the concern and love, 'We keep wondering how Brigid really is. We are so impotent, of course. Poor dear girl. Gladys isn't well and she is very worried about Brigid as we all are. We must continue praying for Brigid . . . The vicar prayed for Brigid.' He was exhausting his supply of cards. 'I must look out for some more. Our desire is, of course, to send to our darling grand-child.' October 15th: 'Andrew's birthday. Brigid just doesn't seem to be responding to treatment and of course we are already suspecting a wrong diagnosis. Such a lovely child and so full of the joy of life.' They had been wanting to see her all this time, but up to now it had been difficult to arrange as Brigie was feeling so unwell. I suggested they came this Friday afternoon: a friend would bring them and they would limit their time with Brigie to half an hour.

Dick wrote: 'We arrived at the post office at two o'clock. Brigid was lovely, but looking a lot more emaciated than when we had last seen her . . . We had a walk round the village, and later joined Jan in a cup of tea: kissed Brigid goodbye and we promised to keep on with the cards for which she thanked us (We didn't know quite what to think.)' On October 20th he wrote: 'Sent a card to Brigid . . . how ill she looked and how impotent we feel regarding her: not knowing what is wrong is the worst thing about it. Prayed for Brigid.' Two days later he was writing: 'Odd how Brigid's T.B. has so upset us both. Jan said she would phone us some day before the weekend to tell us the result of Brigid's operation. It seemed to us oddly ominous that she should quite suddenly have a piece of bone removed and apparently some tissue.'

Brigie would be going back to hospital on Monday and still she had not asked any questions to allow me to be open with her. We hated the pretence, both with her and with other people. As I was getting her ready for sleep that night, she told me that one of our neighbours had talked to her about how worried I had been looking lately, and she was very troubled at the thought. I started to assure her that she did not need to worry about *me*, but in a sudden burst of crying she said, 'And I'm dreading what they're going to tell me at the hospital on Monday. I might have something horrible—like cancer or something.' The word had been spoken. I said, 'They do think you've got a form of cancer, but they don't know what sort. There are many different ones: it could be one that's simple to treat.'

'I bet I've got a bad one. That would be just my luck!' She was quiet for a moment. 'I couldn't die, could I? I *mustn't* die, must I?'

We were not talking about dying, I said. 'We are talking about fighting it.' I told her that her own attitude would be very important: she must be determined to fight it, and we would all be backing her up. She would probably have treatment at a hospital in Leeds.

'Will you come to the hospital every day?'

I told her that of course I would, 'every single day'. We would be behind her helping her to win. Had she been worried about cancer, I asked, without saying anything?

No, she said, she had just thought of it then.

There was another pause.

'I don't think I'll cry again,' she said. 'It was all that worrying and waiting.'

She was calm now, and as she settled down to sleep, burying her head in the pillow, she said, 'I love you, Mum. I think I'll take you with me.' I was very moved: she had never said anything like that to me before. I went out to share the relief that it was in the open with G. As Ruth had said, it might take an 'unfortunate' remark to produce the necessary release and opening.

# 5

––––––––– ⌀ –––––––––

## 'Have you told them what I think?'

*T*he next morning, Brigie and I talked about it more. We talked about our inherited Scottish stubbornness, how it had a good and a bad side, and the good would help her now. She wanted to know who had been told, and I explained that it was only the few who could help at this stage: nobody else should know before she did. I told her about G.M. and Marilyn finding out all they could about treatments, and us all asking advice from people who had experience. We discussed how we should tell the others: Jane and Andrew should be told at home, she thought, 'because then they'll see I'm not scared'. Kate should be told as she would be coming that evening, and Brigie should not have to pretend to anyone. I would go down and see Kate when she got home from work that evening. It all became quite complicated then: we wanted to tell our closest local friends ourselves, and not let them hear the news from anyone else.

There was a problem about Jane. She and Stephen would be talking on the phone during the week, and he would know from Eileen and Colin by then. Once Kate had been told, the whole village would have to know. I decided to ring Jane later on Saturday evening and ask her to come home with Stephen on Sunday, as Brigie 'wanted to see her before she went back to hospital'. She said afterwards that she had been half-expecting a call and thought my reason for her return was 'a bit thin'. I told our neighbour Dorothy that morning, as she was leaving for Bahrain and was very concerned. I met Kate and Steve on their return. We had quite a long talk, and she cried. I told them I wanted to tell people myself, so that they would know we were determined to fight it and to be open about it, and that Brigie was being very strong. I was heartened when Steve said, 'I like the way you're handling this, Janet. I've not seen it done better.' I did not know whether Kate would feel up to coming that evening, but she did and was as perky and cheerful as ever, which was good for Brigie.

On Sunday morning I told Michael. He took the news very quietly, and I talked about the possible treatments and explained why I had not been able to tell him before. He did not ask any questions and I could only hope that his friends would help him to talk about it if he needed to. I saw Eileen and Colin that morning, too, G. talked to Mark, and I went up to Sandra. When I came back Brigie asked me if I'd told her and I said that I had.

'It's just like inviting people to a party, isn't it?' she said. 'Crossing off the names on a list!'

Jane came back in the late afternoon and we went in to Brigie, who had said we should tell her together. Jane wrote about it later:

I got home on Sunday afternoon. I walked into the shop, my mother took me through to Brigie, who was lying on the settee in the sitting room—the room was a sick room, a chair by her side was crowded with medicaments, tissues, half-finished drinks. There were flowers in the room, and a fire burning. My mother told me to sit on the footstool next to Brigie. I started talking, gabbling about what I had been up to, embarrassed, I didn't know how to stop. My mother listened; when a pause came she started, Brigie listened. I had been brought back, she said, so that I could be told at home. Brigie had wanted me to be told at home so I could see that she wasn't frightened. She had cancer.

But we were going to fight it, said Mum, they weren't frightened, and I wasn't to be, because we were all going to fight with Brigie. She was being very strong and brave, and she was going to get better. They didn't know much about it yet, but the results of the tests being carried out on Brigie would come through soon, and then they would know exactly what they had to do to cure it.

I wasn't shocked. I felt very calm, and full of love and respect for Brigie. I seemed to have been prepared for it. Brigie was different again from when I had left her. She was incredibly strong, still retaining some of that distance which made her different. I had been let into one of her secrets. I was sharing a part of her private life, we all were, and this seemed to draw us all together. Brigie had allowed a barrier down. I was privileged, as we all were, and we showed our gratitude by gearing our whole existence towards Brigie.

Brigie had gone pink and looked embarrassed at my praise. Jane seemed calm. I wrote Andrew a stronger letter, trying to prepare him. Both G. and Jane thought it was a bit too strong, but I discovered later in the week that its import had still not reached him. G. decided to ask the office for a week at home and again I was profoundly grateful. We knew that decisions would have to be made soon, and his judgment was invaluable. Jane said she would sleep with Brigie that night; it was good for her to share with her sister, and gave Brigie a rest from my snoring. She decided to stay at home for the week.

In the morning, October 19th, G. and I took Brigie back to Airedale. G. brought the car to the front door, but it was a struggle for Brigie to walk even that far. She found it more comfortable to lie in the back, and put her head on my lap. That way she was less likely to be sick. Jane was looking after the post office for the morning. At the hospital, we went right up to the front door and got a wheelchair. She was put in a single room this time, which she did not like. She caught only

96

a brief glimpse of Clara now and then, taking her creeping steps towards the day room, but by now, I think, she was feeling too sick to enjoy her company anyway. She had her stitches out, a painful procedure which she hated. I saw Dr. Y. in the morning and told him she knew about the cancer. He said they had decided to transfer her to Bradford Royal Infirmary where the chest surgeon, Mr. N., would be able to do a more thorough investigation of her lung. There were no conclusive results as yet from the biopsies of last week. I asked him if the ganglion on her hand had any significance; he was sure it had not. He arranged for me to see the consultant's deputy the next day. We were there all day, taking a break now and then in the refreshment area downstairs when Brigie was being attended to.

A young woman had been admitted to the ward that day and she came in to see Brigie after a while, attracted by the only young face in sight. She told us about the stomach pains that she had been getting and about various trips to the doctor's. After a while she asked Brigie what was wrong with her. I held my breath, wondering how Brigie would cope. She did not hesitate.

'They think I've got cancer,' she said, 'but they're not quite sure.' I do not know what that response did for the young woman's morale, but I rejoiced at Brigie's quick and open answer.

She hated the idea of going to another hospital: she had got used to Airedale now, and was a favourite with many of the staff. It was a bright and modern place and the atmosphere was brisk and cheerful. I tried to say a reassuring word to Clara now and again: she was very anxious about her. When we got back that evening we found that Jane had been busy while we were out. She had given the sitting room a good tidying, but I had a sudden shock when I went in. I had become so used to Brigie being there, and I felt her absence keenly.

On Tuesday morning G. and I had arranged to see Dr. K. and ask his opinion 'off the record' about the standard treatments. He gave us the straight orthodox approach, as our doctor friends had done. If we refused treatment, he said, we would be 'playing with fire'. Ten years ago he himself would not have accepted chemotherapy, but now the treatment was so much more precise, minimising the side-effects. 'There is no treatment that I can recommend outside the N.H.S.'

We went to see Miss Kent and asked her to tell the girls about the diagnosis. We said that Brigie was tackling the illness very positively, that she wanted to see her friends and we hoped they would not be frightened. I offered to talk to them if need be. Somehow we must try to keep everything as normal as possible for her, and her friends were very important. We went back to Litton then: G. would stay at home in the afternoon and I would go to the hospital with Jane.

I met the doctor who was temporarily in charge of the ward there. It was a long consultation, but I do not remember anything about it: in fact there was nothing new to communicate. While I was with him the message came that Brigie should go to B.R.I. the following morning. Did she want to go by ambulance? I asked.

'No,' she said, 'I'd like you and Geoffrey to take me—but I'd like to come back by ambulance.' She needed familiarity going to this strange new place, but was not going to miss the importance of an ambulance journey.

Brigie had other visitors that evening and we came home before her tea. There were always telephone calls to make or answer, and these alone could be very tiring. Her grand-parents still did not know that she had cancer: G.M. thought it best not to tell them before we knew its nature. There were others whose advice I needed: Jane Davies, who was ready to help when we knew precisely about Brigie's cancer and would be able to suggest where the most skilful treatment could be obtained. I had several conversations with her, all very helpful because she had first-hand experience. At some point she asked me whether Brigie had any religious faith, and I said no. In that case, she said, she will take your confidence and assurance, even if death is the outcome. She will take your certainty about another life. That statement was an important support to me, both at the time and later. (Jane Davies and her husband were also very helpful to G.M. and Marilyn in frequent contact and conversation.)

The calls had to be limited to the very essential ones: G. had warned me about the tyranny and the exhaustion that the telephone could bring at such a time, and fortunately all our friends in Herts were getting in touch with G.M. rather than bothering us. Many warming letters were coming, and it was marvellous to know that so many people were thinking about us, but I sensed that some others could not write because they simply did not know what to say. There was a lesson in this for me, remembering times when I, too, had felt lost for the right words: it is better to write one sentence of concern than to remain silent.

That night, when I talked to G.M., he suggested that I relax and watch *Brideshead*: it was a good idea. I could not concentrate on it, but it gave me a respite from the strain.

G. and I got down to Airedale early: I knew Brigie would be feeling very depressed about this next move. Going to a strange hospital was yet another ordeal, and it was useless trying to make bright remarks. I told her that we would ask to stay with her all day, just as we had done at Airedale, and we began, rather drearily, collecting all her cards and the large bunch of flowers that G.M. had sent. The journey was uncomfortable for her, but she lay down in the back most of the way, with her head on my lap.

The reception area at B.R.I. was dreary and crowded; I got a wheelchair for Brigie and during the long wait for her cards I could see her morale sinking very fast. It was uncomfortable for her to sit upright for so long, and she was looking around at the dingy surroundings with great distaste. Even the porters seemed as Dickensian as the building, with no sign of the humour of 'Casanova' who had enlivened her journeys for X-rays at Airedale. At long last, one of them was taking us up to her ward, and at least it was a relief for her to lie down after all this time. She had many unfavourable comparisons to make with Airedale, though: the ward was long and narrow and the line of beds faced a blank partition rather than the windows (possibly just as well because the view, in Brigie's words, was 'just like Wormwood Scrubs'). The bed she found hard and uncomfortable. No one seemed interested in her and her flowers remained in a sink in one of the service rooms. Eventually a nurse came to fill in a form with information that must have been on her records anyway. Simply marking time was demoralising.

G. and I left the ward when they started serving lunch, and I hoped, in our absence, that Brigie would get to know the other two patients who were sitting there in their dressing gowns. They looked pleasant and one was quite young, but they were obviously not going to start talking to Brigie while we were there. For us I hoped there was an equivalent of the pleasant refreshment area at Airedale run by the W.R.V.S., but it turned out to be a very dreary little room with smoking not allowed and nothing to eat but Kit-Kats.

We got back to find that a doctor had been to see Brigie, would do an operation the next day, and wanted an X-ray of her lung and ganglion: we would see him when he had finished that day's operating. Brigie did not like Mr. N., she said. He told her that Airedale had sent her because they were 'so worried' about her, and that idea did not cheer her. She had not mentioned to anyone that she was in pain: the painkiller that she had been given at Airedale before she left was beginning to wear off, and her new pills were not ready yet. She got very distressed when I wanted to ask someone about it. A porter came to take her for an X-ray, and we had to set off without getting any relief. I could only hope that it would not take too long. This was my first experience of a hospital X-ray department, and the hope was not fulfilled.

My heart sank at the sight of a room full of people waiting their turn. There were two X-ray machines but one of them was not functioning properly and people were having to go back two and three times for retakes. Brigie was by now in obvious pain, and again very uncomfortable having to sit upright, but she got very agitated when I wanted to explain this to the sister and ask to jump the queue.

'It always takes as long as this—it did at Airedale,' she said with resignation. 'X-rays usually took about one and a half hours.' It was an insight for me into some of the dreariness that I had not known about. I would have given a great deal then to take her pain myself. We waited there for at least half an hour, probably more, and when she finally went in to the faulty machine I prayed that it would work properly this time, and then we could get her back to her bed quickly. After another wait for the plates to be judged successful, the sister said she would ring for a porter.

Could I not take her back? I asked.

'Oh no, you can't do that. He'll be along in a few minutes.'

The minutes ticked by, and the few became many—another half hour. I could see by the look in Brigie's eyes that she was in distress, but it became even more acute when I begged her to let me ask.

'Don't, Mum, please. We'll just wait.'

Finally the sister came out again.

'Oh, are you still there? I'll give them another ring.' I managed to say that Brigie was in considerable pain and could they please be quick. I cannot remember the explanation of the delay because I felt so agitated at the time. For me it had been the worst experience of all.

When we got back to the ward Brigie was at last given painkillers, and G. went to repark the car. While he was away, a nurse said one of the doctors would see me. I went into an office to meet a quietly spoken, precise man who asked me how much Brigie knew about her illness. I told him that she knew it was cancer, and was prepared to fight it. 'A brave girl,' he remarked. He then took me carefully through every detail of her illness from the beginning, making notes as he did so. I could not imagine what the point of this was: he even wanted to know the names of the T.B. drugs that she had taken. It must have all been in her notes. A nurse came in by mistake when we were about half-way through and I took the chance to ask her to fetch G. The careful notetaking went on after he arrived.

It was suddenly interrupted when the door flew open and a curly haired, round-faced man burst in. Without sitting down or introducing himself, he said to his assistant, 'Have you told them what I think it is?' There was hardly a moment's pause before that rapid, spluttering voice was firing out words of lead.

'It's a sarcoma, starting from that lump on her hand, very rapid, very aggressive and by now widely dispersed through her whole body. It's the only thing that kills girls her age. Boys kill themselves on motorbikes and girls die of this. I'll operate tomorrow and find out definitely, but what I'll have to tell you then will be either awful or bloody awful. The cancer people will take her after the operation, and treatment will be blunderbuss chemotherapy. It's a very rare and aggressive disease, but when you get this trouble in the lung, you look for a lump and there it is. It couldn't be a ganglion: it's in the wrong place, and it's hard.'

I felt as if I'd been turned to stone; again I was staring at the bookshelf behind the younger doctor. When there was a pause I asked the speaker coldly if he was Mr. N.—coldly, because my first feeling was anger. Quite illogically, I wondered how he dared to talk about Brigie like this, to say these appalling things about my daughter, so brutally and harshly. I told him very accusingly that I had promised to tell Brigie 'everything the doctors said': I was blaming him for putting me in this hideous position. I was still angry, in this muddled way, when we left him, but G. said, 'No, it's very good to have frankness after all the flannelling,' and I knew he was right. There was no time to collect our wits: we had to go back and say goodbye to Brigie. It was a mercifully short stop, though, as Jane and Stephen were coming to see her during the visiting hour.

I do not know how G. managed to drive us home that night, but he did. I felt too stunned even to cry, but the tears came at last and gave some relief. G. stopped at a pub and we had a drink, but we could not stay long as loud music started, and that was unbearable. We were coming into Skipton and G. said, 'I know we don't feel like it but we have got to eat.' He bought fish and chips and we had them in a lay-by: it was like mechanically stoking up an engine and just as cheerless. It was as it had been on that other night of shock: an outside person, quite separate from me, it seemed, had to talk to Michael when we got home. We told him about Brigie's operation the following day, but nothing about the significance of it: I had to get myself in order before I could do that. When he went to bed G. offered to ring G.M. I was grateful. I was in no state to do it. It was very difficult for G. and he cried while he was talking, for which, quite unnecessarily, he felt ashamed. He rang again later, when he felt calmer, suggesting that they come up the next day. We would have some agonising decisions to make about treatment. Jane and Stephen came back and we tried to be normal, but they both knew, it seems, that something was wrong.

I had long spells that night, trying to be quiet in myself. I reread one or two of the letters of support, especially the ones from Fairacres. 'Suffering and death for the young is a mystery,' wrote the now retired Mother Mary Clare, 'but He is love, and has riches in store for you all. That sounds pious platitudes . . .' No one who had ever met Mother Mary Clare would ever associate pious platitudes with her: the words carried the authority of a life devoted to self-giving love. The Sisters of the Love of God at Fairacres give the most full and unconditional love to all that I have ever experienced. Mother Jane had said, 'In all the anguish and agony for you, there's nothing one can say to "help". All we can do is to love and pray and ask you to "lean" on us.' I was leaning very heavily that night, a time of extreme weakness and turmoil, and I knew the support would somehow hold me up. There were other letters which helped too, especially those that expressed confidence in me facing the challenge in the right way. These were the two elements, I realised later, that gave me strength: the awareness of the support of prayer and love, and the confidence and warmth of friends who believed in our capacity to cope.

One other thing became clear during the night. I could no longer bear Andrew to be apart from all this. He did not even know that Brigie had cancer, and now that events were moving so quickly he must be told. I would ring him in the morning, Thursday, and ask him to come home at once, not wait for the weekend. G. suggested that he come to Bradford and get a taxi to the hospital. Andrew was very surprised to get my call—the second letter, too, had failed to alert him—but he readily agreed to leave at once. He would ring Jane during the day and tell her what time he would reach Bradford, as I wanted to meet him outside the hospital. She had, by now, been told what Mr. N. had said and was going to stay in the post office (G. and I wanted to leave early and be with Brigie before the operation) but I thought it was too hard to leave her alone after hearing this news. I rang Ruth and asked her to come up: together they finished making the damson jam that I had been unable to deal with.

Brigie was more pleased than usual to see us that morning. She kept saying, 'I'm really glad you're here, you know': she was always nervous before the injection of the pre-med and it seemed a long morning of waiting for her. Hers was to be the last of the morning's operations. A photographer had taken a picture of her hand with the 'ganglion': Mr. N. wanted it for lecture purposes. Brigie felt quite important: 'What a pity it's my hand with the wart on,' she said. She was feeling better about the hospital too: someone had arranged her flowers for her and she was settling down. It was good that G.M. and Marilyn got there before she had her pre-med, and as the hospital allowed only two visitors at a time we took it in turns to be with her until she went into the theatre. Marilyn remembers they had a long talk together, and Brigie told her how good she felt with Jane now.

The four of us went back to the car and had the sandwiches and coffee we had brought from home. There was nothing we could do for an hour or two until Brigie came back to the ward. The sister had said not to return until about 3 or 4 p.m., so there was time to talk and see how we all felt about treatment. We all hated the thought of it, but if it could possibly save Brigie's life, would we have a choice? At this stage, we simply did not have enough information and would have to talk to Mr. N. about it. During the afternoon I met him in the corridor and said that we were very doubtful about this blunderbuss chemotherapy and he said, 'There is a case for refusing it.' He would get a friend of his from Cookeridge Hospital to come the next day and talk to us about it. 'He's a very wise old man,' he said. Mr. N. was somewhat puzzled about the family. 'We thought we'd talked to the parents last night,' he said, 'and then these other people turned up.' He was obviously reluctant at first to talk to more than two people, and we did not want to irritate him. However, by next day he seemed to have adapted.

Andrew was going to arrive at about three thirty, and I waited for him in the forecourt, very nervous about what I had to say. The others were up near the ward, and I wanted to be there when Brigie woke up. I took Andrew to the car and gave him the remnants of our lunch: I told him that Brigie had cancer and that the doctor here thought it was 'pretty bad'. I thought that was enough for him to cope with at the moment. We had a cry together, and went up to the ward. I had warned Andrew that Brigie would look very ill after her operation and while recovering from the anaesthetic, and indeed she did, breathing heavily and noisily through the oxygen mask, but she knew Andrew and smiled. She knew enough, too, to replace the oxgyen mask when her coughing disturbed it, but she was asleep most of the time, just having sips of water from time to time. We stayed until the end of the visiting hour, when all was being made ready for the night, and came back to Litton for a meal. Michael was up at Sandra's and G. went up to collect him.

G. had only just gone when the phone rang. It was a long and complicated call from a neighbour of G.'s elderly father in Sheffield; his problems were again becoming unmanageable. I was still talking to her when G. got back and he took over. It was almost too much after that day. G. rang his daughter Helen and asked her if she would go and sort things out. His first priority was here. I think Val had made us a large pie, and it was very heartening to have tasty and hot food after the strain of the day. This kind of thoughtfulness helped to keep us going: there was no time to cook, but we had to eat and everyone was getting tired of the fish and chips that we had collected so many times on the way back from the hospital.

The next day, Friday, G. would look after the post office and do the balance. G.M. would take Marilyn to Leeds (she had to go back to London for the day) and Jane, Andrew and I would go to the hospital. G.M. would join us there. Brigie was recovering from the operation, and she liked Mr. N. now, she said, even though he had told her the cancer was bad. 'It's a big one,' he had said. But he had also said she could come home soon, and she liked him for that—and it would be by ambulance. G.M. arrived and gave her two pretty new nighties. The nurses took off her operation gown and dressed her in the pink one, and her morale improved. There was a problem with her pulse rate, though, and she was put on a monitoring machine. We took turns sitting with her.

I remember [Jane wrote] knowing the best place to sit was the good hand side, the one which was free of bandages. The day after her operation I was very moved when I came to take my turn with Brigie, who was lying very uncomfortably on her side, bolstered by five or six pillows, struggling to breathe. She acknowledged that I was there, and then drifted into sleep again. Dad was sitting holding her hand, with her face towards him. She woke up a while later and asked Dad if I was still there, as she could not see me behind her. He said I was, and she moved her bandaged hand across her body for me to hold.

When we were not with Brigie we would trail about those cheerless corridors and stairways or go out for a cigarette on the front steps, where the autumn wind was blowing the leaves about among the cars. The dying time of the year, I remember thinking, and all the time there was the overriding worry about how I was going to talk to Brigie about her own death. I knew I had to be honest with her: I had promised that, and it was the only way for her, I was sure. Looking back afterwards, Jane remembered that one day in the hospital at this stage Brigie had asked where I was. When Jane told her that I had gone out for a cigarette Brigie had remarked, 'She'll need a cigarette soon!' The periods away from the ward meant that we had time to talk to each other, and during that day Jane told Andrew the details of what Mr. N. had said to us on Wednesday night. Michael and Nigel Dagett had asked to come that night, but Brigie was still very sleepy after the operation and not well enough to see friends, we thought. Andrew offered to ring them and explain. I had muddled the visiting rota, though, and Pat and Joanne arrived. We suggested that they stay just a short time, and Jane went in with them.

In the late afternoon the specialist arrived from Cookeridge Hospital and he and Mr. N. talked to G.M. and me with Jane and Andrew in the corridor. It was very informal: he seemed very humane and anxious to help. He had not seen Brigie but he had looked at the plates. His blue eyes travelled round the group, and looking at me he said, gently and firmly, 'No treatment—it wouldn't be kind.' There was nothing he could do to save her life, and treatment could give only distress. He went in with Mr. N. to see Brigie and came out even graver. She had weeks rather than months, he said. It was a question of keeping her comfortable and providing us with all we needed to nurse her at home. I asked his advice about how to tell her she was dying.

'You mustn't let her give up hope,' he said. 'I've taken young doctors right through to the end without their realising they were dying. It can be done.' Mr. N. said nothing. I was less happy about this: surely it would not be right to be dishonest with Brigie? And yet he was a wise and experienced doctor. His opinion would have to be considered. I had read about the 'conspiracy of silence' which can happen in families, where the dying member wants to talk but keeps silent for fear of causing pain. Facing death in loneliness and separation must be avoided for Brigie.

I wondered how Jane and Andrew had coped with this straight, explicit talk, especially Andrew who had been suddenly thrust into the crisis so recently. An answer to this question came later in the evening when I was serving a meal at home. Michael and Andrew had gone off somewhere, and at last Jane went to find them. She came back a few minutes later and beckoned me to come. I went out to the kitchen to one of the closest family moments of the whole time. Jane had found them sitting together outside the barn, Andrew's arm round Michael and both crying. She brought them in. Andrew's arm was still round Michael, whose head was slumped in grief. I realised what had happened. We, simply, the four of us, held on to each other in a very close circle for a long few moments. Words were not necessary, but I remember saying at last, 'I think I'm very lucky having four such marvellous kids' ( Jane said, 'We've got a marvellous Mum') 'and we're all going to stay very close and hold on to each other, and look after each other, especially the youngest.' It was like that for a long time until the need for tissues broke the circle. Jane and I told them it was good to cry and they must not think it was unmanly. G. came in a few minutes later, and agreed, and told them how he had cried about Brigie.

When I asked Andrew later why he had decided to tell

Michael that Brigie was going to die, he said he did not think it right that everyone but Michael knew, and he did not see why I had to do the telling every time. Andrew had lived through a great deal of experience in just two days, and had grown.

It was a very adult decision.

# 6

---❧---

## The good week

We gave it this name, because in many ways, in spite of the pain, it was a time of great happiness. Brigie was home again surrounded by overwhelming proof of her importance to a great many people, and there was a new quality in her which made us all want to be with her. The greatest hardship for anyone during this time and later was for those who had to be absent. It was a solace to sit quietly in that room, holding her hand or just looking at her when she was asleep, wondering about the dreams that brought a smile to her face and unintelligible remarks to her lips. She was busy about many matters, we felt, when she was sleeping: there was an other-worldly quality there which one longed to share. But the smile when she woke up was earthly again as she returned to the realm of friends and events. It was a busy time for us, a perpetual round of answering the phone to many friends, arranging visits, making endless cups of coffee, keeping the household fed and the clothes washed and seeing that Brigie was not getting too tired. She could always drift off into sleep, though, and join in the conversation again when she woke up, or she could ask for the bedpan, a sure way of emptying the room. It was the school's half-term holiday, and many of her friends from Skipton were able to come, as well as those from the South. They were the ones who saw most clearly the remarkable change in her.

That Saturday morning when Brigie was to come home by ambulance G. took me to Bradford so that I could travel with her. Soon after we arrived the physiotherapist came in to give her exercises to do at home. I have a vivid picture of her sitting up in bed in her new nightie, her face tense and pink with the concentration needed for following the instructions for leg and arm exercises in spite of the discomfort from her stitches. She did not need any of the jollying encouragements that other patients did: she was giving all she had. I took note of how the physio held her to ease the coughing and relieve the phlegm. Mr. N. came in: he was not on duty, but I had the feeling that there were not many days when he did not check on his ward. He had prescribed pills to regulate the pulse and strong painkillers that had a sedative effect so that she should not need sleeping pills as well.

'Get all her pals in,' he said. 'Plenty of friends around her. And don't let her sleep too much in the day, then she'll be better at night.' He went into a long explanation of how our internal clock does not work well for the sick, and day and night can become confused. They were getting on splendidly now, the doctor and the patient. He never called her by her name. She was always 'Gorgeous' or 'Smart', and she loved it. She told me that he had shouted out loudly one day across the barrier to the men's section: 'Anyone over there want a gorgeous girl? We've got an absolute smasher over here!' There was a palliative operation, he told us privately, that he might do if her pulse rate settled down: he could open her chest and remove the obstruction to improve her breathing. It was a major operation, and he would have to weigh up the advantages to her breathing with 'the pain in her side' which it would give her, and whether, in fact, she had enough time to benefit from the surgery. I should ring him the following Wednesday and report progress. The district nurse would come and the G.P. ('Those Dales doctors are a special breed,' he said). He would have her back at any time if we could not cope.

It was a pleasant surprise to find that we would travel in the Grassington ambulance with the drivers who had called to see us on the day we moved into the post office—Brian and David. They were splendid, taking great pains to make sure that Brigie was in the right position. 'We've got to have you comfortable, pet.' There was no unnecessary fuss but, in between jobs, lots of jokes. As we travelled we heard their version of the journey to Airedale with Dennis the year before, now enshrined in dale lore as events involving Dennis almost invariably are. Brigie enjoyed that: it made her feel as if she was on home ground already. It was a great moment for Brigie when we came into the dale. 'We're in Littondale, Brigie, and it's raining.' 'Typical,' she said happily. I had a sudden thought that this might be the last time she came up this road and had to make myself think of something else very quickly. I must not cry.

There was a large group in the sitting room to welcome her home, everyone smiling and happy. The fire was on and the pillows ready. Brian and David thought they should be taking her up to bed, but this was where she wanted to be. They would lift her very gently on to the settee, and made careful plans.

'You put your arms right round my neck, pet, and then we won't hurt you.'

As she did so she said coyly to Brian, 'We can't go on meeting like this', and her audience loved it. What a relief to know that Brigie was still herself.

We all had coffee and fruit cake (Mrs. Yeadon's, I think) and the others heard a repetition of the anecdote about Dennis. Jane saw Sandra setting off to walk to Halton Gill and brought her in to get a lift. I was glad that Sandra saw Brigie then: she would know there was nothing frightening. Brian and David left, and quite suddenly Brigie said, 'I'm really happy now that I'm home. I'm really happy now.' There was that ringing tone in her voice and the look on her face which told us that those emphatic words were true. We had our lunch after that, potato soup yet again, I think, all in the sitting room with Brigie, someone perching on the settee end. It was the first of many such meals, some very quiet when Brigie was sleeping or very ill, but this relaxed and cheerful, a very happy reunion. People were in and out all day. G.M., Marilyn and Andrew went up the hill in the afternoon to see that Shez's blanket was still in place and to take Sam for a walk. Mark and Kate came in the evening with lovely presents for Brigie. Kate gave her a beautiful white broderie-anglaise nightie and a white dressing gown that she and Steve had chosen during the day, and Mark brought out a dainty gold signet ring. 'It's gold,' he had told his mother; 'only the best is good enough for Brigie.' She was thrilled. It was a perfect fit, thanks to Kate's advice, and he would take it to be engraved with her initials.

Brigie was tired after all this excitement: perhaps, I hoped, she would manage to sleep through my snoring.

On Sunday, G.M. and Marilyn would go to see his parents: they still did not know that Brigie had cancer. Dick's diary entry for October 24th says:

. . . The phone rang and Geoffrey, who is in Yorkshire, told me he is up seeing Brigid and would call on us tomorrow to talk to us about Brigid's condition. She is very ill he said—asked us not to prepare any special lunch. We fear what he is going to tell us. [Of the next day he wrote] Brigid is suffering from a virulent form of cancer. This awful news was brought by Geoffrey this morning for in response to his promise Geoffrey arrived just after noon to tell of the sad talk they had with the Bradford cancer specialist . . . We were shattered by this news and spent the rest of the day near tears. We won't get used to it I'm sure, for however much people assure us of Brigid's fortitude and courage, we shall know, at the back of our minds, and be conscious that we shall never again see that vivacious lovely person who is Brigid but what we shall see is one for whom we shan't be able to hide our sympathy. Geoffrey left early for he is hoping to get back and home before nightfall . . . So, after he had gone, what could one say? We both seemed unable to carry on a reasonable conversation—for it is odd how this kind of news attacks one. I suppose it is something to do with the inevitability of it and our not being able to do anything. A very miserable evening—we solaced ourselves as best we could, at home.

In Litton, Brigie was having her first visit from Sister D. She came in warm and gusty and full of encouraging chat. I got what she needed and left her with Brigie, who still liked her privacy. Brigie felt much more comfortable after a wash and a clean nightie. It was very good for us to know that we would have this professional help every day. I was managing the bedpan routine, with Brigie lifting herself up on her elbows, but it was useful to see the expert arranging the pillows and showing us how to move her more easily and comfortably. She told me much later that she and Sister N. were very unsure about what they would find with this 'case' and that she was preparing herself mentally as she came up the dale for what she thought might be a very difficult situation. It was a shock, she acknowledged a year later, to be suddenly confronted that day with Brigie as she came through the front door: she had expected at least a few minutes' conversation with the rest of the family before she met her patient. It was the first of many highly unconventional circumstances. That day, however, her large presence did not give any impression of uncertainty and Brigie liked her bracing approach. She and Jane discussed afterwards how they would describe her and decided she was jolly.

For lunch that day G. had made Brigie's favourite topside with mushrooms and she managed to eat a little. In the afternoon, Gumby rang and asked if he could come and see Brigie. She was very pleased to see him again. G.M. and

Marilyn returned from Lancs. They would have a meal and then set off for Broxbourne, taking Jane back with them and Andrew for his train to Bangor. We felt they should both try to live normal lives—we did not know how long this would go on and Andrew had only just started his course. Brigie had loved her weekend with them—she was to talk about it later—but she would surely wonder and be alarmed if everyone stayed. Jane described her feelings as they went over the Barks road and looked down the dale . . . 'I could just pick out our tiny house, in the midst of our small village, within which something very big and someone very important was lying.'

In the evening Michael and Nigel Dagett came with the first of Margaret's marvellous bakes, a supreme example of kindness. It was a huge carton of cakes, biscuits, pies and flans, all neatly packed in plastic bags, and included even the wire twists in case we wanted to put them in the freezer. Their mother, I discovered later, was only three weeks out of hospital herself. There were presents for Brigie, too—a comical soft character with immensely long legs which he hugged in his arms. He was from Helen, and he sat on the settee back to Brigie's great delight. She called him Pete. There were flowers, too, and a honeycomb. It was a lovely evening for Brigie.

G. went back to London on Monday morning. He had been home now for two weeks, and we would miss him. When he got there he realised that he simply could not stay away from home. He was in the office for one hour and came straight back, having arranged to work from here. So for that day, Brigie and I were the only ones in the household, but she had many visitors. Peggy came first with Karen and her eleven-month-old Nicola. It was marvellous to see Brigie's pleasure, holding out her arms for the baby.

'Oh, you've come to see me, you little love,' and her eyes shone. The little thing sat on her tummy for ages, very quietly. I was worried that it would be uncomfortable for

Brigie, who was very distended with fluid, but she would not let the baby go, and the child was happy, too. We all had coffee and Margaret's oat biscuits. Another visitor arrived: Margaret Walker with a beautiful arrangement of plants for Brigie—a present from the village. The card said that they were all looking forward to the time when Brigie would come flying out the door again in the morning for her lift to school—toast in hand as always! Jack, our postman, joined the group and she liked his jokes. It was the beginning of the almost perpetual party of that week. I lost count of how many people dropped in for a few moments or longer. The professionals would have been aghast if they had known quite how many people came, but I am convinced that it was good for Brigie.

On that Monday afternoon Sister N. came for the first time; she was quieter than Sister D. but Brigie had a good first impression. She came every day that week, and several times she had some very helpful talks with us. She told me, one day, that Brigie had asked her if she saw many people who were dying. I asked her where the emphasis came in that question. If it came on the word 'many', we would know that Brigie was further ahead than we realised, but she could not be sure. Even so, the fact that Brigie had asked such a question must mean something. Brigie had gone on to say to the nurse, 'But I'm not going to die. I'm fighting—and I've got my family to back me up.' She had dreams, however, about dying: one was about Dr. Y. coming to the house and telling her that she would have to go back to hospital and die. When she told me I could only say, 'Oh, Brigie!' Perhaps I should have asked her, I thought later, about how she felt when he said that, but I had not been ready at the time. G. came back in the early evening. 'Oh Geoffrey, Geoffrey,' Brigie said with intense pleasure as he sat holding her hand. He was to say later that the only person who could cheer him during this time was Brigie herself. She was giving us all much love and gratitude, and her delight when Jane rang to say that *she* was coming back the next day

116

was extreme. Jane has described that day she spent in London:

That morning is now a blur of faces and memories or things said. I wanted to talk about it all, to tell people, just to pour it all out repeatedly. I also needed to tell tutors—they had to know the uncertainty which I would be working under—I might not be there for very long. It seemed very strange, talking about all this in corridors and stairways. I felt I was not really there totally, the part of me which was wandering around, unable to settle down to think about work, was merely the shell of myself, the best part of me was with Brigie and Mum in our home in that small village.

It was a marvellous feeling to know that she would be back. She had been so thoughtful and good to talk to during the previous week. When G. said 'I do think it's right that Jane should be here,' I knew I had misjudged it: nothing, not even her course, was more important than what was going on here. He joked with her when she got back, 'Well, you managed to stay away longer than I did.'

Mark and Kate came that evening. She gave Brigie her little bear which Brigie had always liked. There were even more visitors the next day. Margaret Dagett came in the morning and then Val. They stayed to lunch. It was Alison in the afternoon. She had brought Chris from London to see her friend during her half-term, and Brigie was very pleased. Alison would ride Shez and bring her round for Brigie to see. There had been some discussion about Shez: the weather was getting colder and I knew we could not look after her while Brigie was ill. Mark's mother had rung some time ago very upset to hear that Brigie had cancer and offering to take Shez for the winter. It was a very helpful suggestion. Brigie was happy: Shez would be well looked after and Mark's sisters would ride her. When we learned, though, that Brigie might have only a short time we did not want

Shez to go so far away; at least Brigie should be able to see her. It was still impossible to share these thoughts with anyone outside the family: we had to prevaricate about Shez.

Janet and Abigail, from school, came that afternoon, and another furry animal joined the line on the settee back: this was Floyd, the yellow dog. When Eileen and Colin were in later, Brigie made the remark that he would relate many times later on. Looking at all her animals and the other presents and flowers, she said with a sparkle, 'Aren't I lucky?' Robert and Angela came over from Kirkby Lonsdale, and in the evening all her friends from the gift shop: Mary Ann and Jenny, Mrs. S. and Pauline. They all brought more presents for her and for us, and Mark and Kate were there too. Brigie was very tired at the end of it all, but it was a super day for her and she loved all this attention and concern. Jane had brought her Joe, her own favourite bear. She would sleep with Brigie that night and give her a rest from my snoring, calling me if she wanted the bedpan.

The bond between the sisters, developing during the previous week, now grew and flourished. All the old rivalries were forgotten, and as if to symbolise it Jane had given Brigie the bangle that they had squabbled about for years. They seemed to enter into a fresh area together, delighting in a new and adult awareness of each other, concentrating into these few weeks a lifetime of love and closeness. As Marilyn was to say later, 'It was like watching a love affair develop.' Jane became very sensitive to Brigie's needs, knowing when she was getting tired, or her spirits were flagging, able to tell me when it was time to move people on. This eased the load for me immeasurably, and became more important as the good week went on.

The day after Jane came back, Wednesday, was an even more chaotic one. Chris and Katie came in the morning with Alison, who later went up to see the farrier reshoe Shez. Rebecca from Westhill Road was coming for lunch with her parents and brother, Anthony. It was lovely for Brigie but I knew it was going to be a hectic day. Gayna and other friends were coming in the afternoon—it was their only opportunity. I was in the kitchen when these other five visitors poured through the front door into the sitting room and Marion, Rebecca's mother, told me how Brigie had taken charge and introduced everybody, keeping the conversation going with this very mixed group. It all seemed very muddly to me, but Marion wrote later about the calm and serene atmosphere and I was reassured by that. Later still, she recorded her impressions of that day:

On Wednesday, October 28th, during the half-term stay with Anthony in Out Gate, we drove to Litton on a damp, grey day to visit Brigie. We arrived at about midday and were warmly welcomed by Janet, Geoffrey, Jane and Brigie who was lying on the settee in a room overflowing with flowers and cards. 'It looks like a shop, doesn't it,' said Brigie. She looked lovely, sitting propped up among the cushions with her hair curling over her shoulders, and was evidently pleased to see us. She said, 'Tell me all the news,' which we tried to do, talking about the changes in Hoddesdon and Westhill Road, about Rachel in Africa and our own recent activities in the Lake District and on the C.N.D. march in London. Rebecca gave Brigie a woolly lamb which she instantly named Larry and he was put with a row of Snoopies she had along the back of the settee. Brigie was so gay and lively and interested in everything that she made one forget how ill she was and what discomfort she was suffering. She looked very pretty with shining eyes and hair and yet with an ethereal quality that was very moving.

  Soon after we arrived she was visited by some school friends and the room was filled to overflowing. Jan gave us a delicious soup for lunch which Brigie enjoyed too and we talked about the sort of foods she fancied. We left her then to talk to her friends and then the doctor and nurse arrived to see her. Afterwards although she was tired and drifted off to sleep for short spells, Rebecca sat holding her hand and Jane brushed her hair. She said, 'You are good to me, Jane.' To which Jane replied, 'And you are good to me too,' and we saw the wonderfully close bond that had grown up between them and realised that they had been privileged to know a closeness and depth of understanding that few sisters achieve even when they [are] together and know each other over many long years.

When Brigie dozed she seemed to be in some vivid world from which she returned smiling with the questions, 'Have I been asleep, what did I say?' She was very sweet in her concern for others and apologised to Rebecca because Shez was lame and couldn't be ridden. 'I hope when you come at Christmas you can ride her,' she said.

It was very hard to drag ourselves away although we knew Brigie must be tired but in spite of the intense sorrow of knowing we should probably not see her again we were also uplifted by the great sense of love in the house and a wonderfully positive feeling that Brigie's indomitable spirit and lovely, warm personality would be with us and inspire us always.

Anthony, too, wrote his account of their visit in his diary. 'If you think Jan would like it then send her this copy,' he wrote to his mother. 'It is agonising not being able to express what one wants but I think it goes a little way to describe the way I felt and thought that day. It wasn't written for anybody and for no reason other than that I find I must write things down, maybe in order to understand them properly.' This is his record:

Monday, 2nd November, 1981. Wednesday as I have already written was a day we looked forward to with uncertainty, and I at least with a degree of fear. Until the evening before I hadn't decided if I would join the others (rather than 'would' I should probably write 'could'). It proved however to be a day that although very sad was also so full of love I was happy and proud to be a part of it . . . Litton is a beautiful dale, less crowded than most. Everywhere was grey through a faint mist and slight drizzle. It all felt, strangely, even more like being in the country than the Lake District does. We walked into the post office and the expected shambles. The P.O. itself is very small and cluttered with posters, leaflets, postcards and some provisions. Paper seems to be everywhere. From the P.O. the stairs run up to the first floor of the cottage and a corridor leads to the kitchen and living room downstairs. We were led into the kitchen—full of disorder and people. Mugs are on back numbers of the *Guardian*, half-read novels are amongst the dishes. It is impossible to open the door because of a mass of boots and Barbour jackets. From this chaos Jan is able to conjure wonderful meals with apparently little effort. The supply of tea and coffee can only be rivalled by that consumed by the characters of *Dallas*. And while all this is going on inside, outside the window the side of the dale rises steeply to the grey leaden sky, taking up a line of walls and displaying magically the outcropping of weathered rocks. And it all frames a gushing stream which emerges from the middle of the hill. Up there somewhere is Brigie's horse—Shez.

We spent the morning with Brigie talking to her and amongst ourselves. Some school friends of hers also visited, and everybody seemed to have brought some cuddly toy. These were instantly named and sat in line on the back of the sofa on which poor Brigie lay. Bright and outwardly cheerful she lay there without even the strength to sit up and reach for a drink. Apart from this she seemed well, except when she had short bouts of coughing. She knows she has cancer (hell, that was a hard word to write) and knows what the result will almost certainly mean, and is still somehow able to be bright, and cheerfully comment on her surprise at how nice people have been. 'I thought they would have taken the opportunity to put me in a dark corner and forget me,' she says with a sparkling laugh. We look at her and smile a little—certainly a genuine smile but it hides held-back tears. She must somehow be experiencing a happiness none of us can really understand. But what we can feel is the love. Never before have I felt so much of it—that at least will always maintain the bonds with Brigie and is why we felt no despair in the room.

Rebecca sat on the sofa with Brigie and held her hand while we all talked and had a drink. Somehow Jan managed to produce a lovely dinner of soup followed by oat cakes, fruit loaf and more coffee. She said that everybody in the village had been wonderfully helpful providing food and other things to save Jan and the family more time to spend with Brigie. After lunch Mum helped by doing the washing up while the rest of us went for a short walk with Jane. Even though (or perhaps because) it was a dull grey day the dale looked beautiful, far more simplistic than the Lakes, no trees or towering hills to break the skyline, only walls and outcrops of rock seem to interrupt the green grey grass of the steep slopes. We crossed the river while Jane told stories of how quickly it rises and falls, changing in minutes from a dry bed to a raging torrent. And then down a muddy path to see Dennis—the local farmer and character. He was hard at work, with Michael's help, clipping the ewes for tupping and giving them the winter dip. Michael was working very hard and had clearly settled well into country Yorkshire life—he has also developed a very respectable accent. When it began to rain we made our way back via Brigie's horse. Rebecca adjusted her blanket but she didn't seem greatly interested.

On getting back to the cottage we sat again in the room with Brigie. Rebecca held her hand while she dozed off to a dreamy sleep making strange mumbling sounds and uttering unintelligible words. Something about going upstairs to get some cheese. Dad and I sat in silence. I looked at the beautiful and peaceful face on the sofa and thought of the happy bouncing girl of Westhill Road. Not for the first time that day my eyes glazed over. And they do again now as I write these pages, and the same images pass through my mind. They aren't tears of grief and despair so much as of wonder and love which especially during periods of silence is so strong in that cottage, and so warm.

We left shortly after this and made our way back to Out Gate in the dark. Little was said on the journey—probably because we all had deep feelings and things we wanted to say but knew we could not express them adequately and without making them sound trivial and planned. All I know is that somehow seeing Brigie and her loving family gave me strength and not despair. However little hope there may be there is still a small crack (and always will be) through which we can grasp, be it for a miracle or some other strength . . . I spend a lot of time thinking of Brigie and praying. She may never know it but she's changed me.

On November 10th he wrote to his mother:

I will send Brigie another card in the next day or so. I think about her a lot and pray a good deal too. Rachel found a spiritual strength on an African plateau. I for some reason I cannot explain have found it in Brigie and her family. For the first time in a long time I feel that a prayer of some kind may help. Maybe it's that we didn't realise before how much we love Brigie, and maybe it's more.

It must have been very difficult for them all to say goodbye, especially for Rebecca. Her father had told her everything and she had been terribly upset. 'But Brigie's my best friend,' she had said. I thought she managed very well that day: they were all able to say goodbye to Brigie cheerfully, but they had to get away very quickly afterwards.

Sandra and Jean came later, on their way back from the ante-natal clinic at Airedale. 'I can't wait till Sandra has her baby,' Brigie had been saying for weeks. A furry owl joined the Snoopies that Val and the girls had brought. Kate and Mark were there as always. We counted up and she had eighteen visitors that day.

The doctor would have been shocked, I'm sure, if he had known about it. It was the senior doctor coming all this week as Dr. K. was away. We wondered if this was a diplomatic absence because he was embarrassed about his wrong diagnosis at the beginning, and G. made a point of telling his colleague that we had appreciated Dr. K.'s help earlier and asked him to say so. He confirmed that these cancers are incredibly difficult to catch in time. Even a doctor's son that he knew of, with every possible treatment, had still died. He was very impressed with Brigie. 'I keep asking her for complaints,' he said, 'and I can't get one.' He was in touch with Mr. N. about the possibility of a palliative operation, 'a potentially lethal operation', he called it, even though Brigie's condition had improved considerably in the last few days. When I spoke to him Mr. N. wanted to know about her breathing, and I discovered that G. had been timing it, so we were able to tell him. They said it was still too early to decide, and Brigie was relieved that her return to hospital was postponed. The doctor gave us a prescription for diamorphine which we were very reluctant to have, but he said he wanted us to have it in the house in case we needed it. When G. took the prescription to Skipton he had much difficulty. The first three chemists had none, and the fourth insisted on ringing the doctor to make sure that it was in order to dispense it. At the same time G. bought some Complan and Carnation Build-up in the hope that we could encourage Brigie to take some nourishment.

By Thursday the excitement and momentum of coming home to flowers and friends in streams was beginning to lessen. As Jane said, we had stopped talking about fighting the illness and nothing was happening about treatment.

Mark was asking pointed questions and what was Brigie thinking? Her morale was flagging and so was mine, I realised. I seemed to be losing my rapport with her and not giving her what she needed. Physical tiredness was one factor, but I realised that I was thinking too much about her dying and had become quiet and withdrawn. Brigie needed buoyancy around her, not shallow bounciness, but 'quietness and confidence'. Jane had this and Brigie turned to her, making me feel both guilty and inadequate. I remembered what Maurice had said about her need to take strength from us: that we would have to be resource-full people in order to help her. I would have to shake myself out of this emotional lethargy, looking at the thing from Brigie's point of view and not letting my own feelings get in the way.

Jane spent a lot of time with her and they had long conversations about the animals. Another Snoopy, from Stephen, had joined in: there was 'Soppy Snoopy' and 'Junior Snoopy'. Jane wrote:

We talked a great deal in that week, she and I. We discovered all the things I had wanted to talk with her about, not important in their own right, but as a way of sharing each other's views and opinions. I felt I wanted to tell her some of the things which meant something to me, we played her favourite songs on the record player, and I described what it was like to be able to make a drawing especially for somebody, and regretted not having the time to make one for her. Instead I put an old drawing of mine up on the wall for her to look at among the flowers and Christmas cactus, combed her hair when she was feeling comfortable, and shaped her nails. She amazed me one day when she said she had always wanted to do my hair, and sat on the settee, weak as she was, and put it in pigtails. I left them in all day and showed customers in the shop, so proud I was to be wearing Brigie's pigtails.

They would also write Andrew a letter in colour: Jane would write and draw and Brigie would hold the pencils and suggest colours and ideas. The project helped Brigie over many a dull time, and kept her spirits up. Visitors were still coming, but not as many. Jane would often stay with them, and she could tell me when Brigie had grown tired or was finding someone trying. People did not always give Brigie what she needed. She said after one visit, 'She wasn't very nice to me today. She didn't kiss me or hold my hand.' She needed the physical contact. 'What a waste of time' after another: there had not been any real communication. We had to balance people's need to see Brigie with the pleasure it gave her or with her tolerance for them. 'Well, I've got to see them some time, haven't I?' was one resigned acceptance, and, 'Do you think you can be there when they come, so that you can change the subject?' One thing she did hate was discussion of medical details. Nor did people invariably make valuable suggestions to me. Most would ask what would be helpful for us or for Brigie: there were one or two who thought they knew best and pressed a totally inappropriate idea. Once this was actually hurtful in its thoughtlessness.

Brigie thought it an honour that Dennis would come with Val one evening. G. gave him several whiskies with lemon and the anecdotes flowed. Brigie loved it, but her eyes would roll with tiredness from time to time, and she would drift away. 'Now it's like this, you see, Brigid,' he said, and she would be with him again, laughing at the colourful language and the punch-line of his story. More girls came afterwards, and one of their mothers. One group had to make way for the next. On Friday she and Jane did more work on the letter during the morning, which was usually her best time. G. carefully and illegally date-stamped it for them with our Litton postmark. It was not actually going in the post, as Andrew had rung to say he was coming home at the weekend and he would have it then. They were both very pleased with the completed task.

# Dear Andrew

## From Brigie + Jane

The flow of visitors in the household has decreased slightly today so we now have time to write you a note. We are being watched by eight cuddly toys + one pottery hedgehog. They consist of: SNOOPY, LARRY, JOE, PETE, THOMAS, JUNIOR-SNOOPY, LUCKY OWL, SOPPY-SNOOPY, + FRED the hedgehog.

Hope you're not still swooning over Lady Di! I bet there's loads of fit pieces down there - BRIGIE said that, not Jane. BRIGIE has just been put on a sheepskin rug. by the nurse she keeps calling the mid-wife.

This is Brigie ⟶

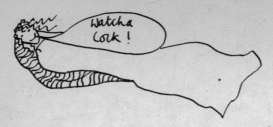

It is like Interflora in the sitting-room, there are CARNATIONS, CHRYSANTHUMUMS, CHRYSANTHAMUMS, FERNS, TIGER LILIES, and CACTUS. MICHAEL will be ¡¡SOAKED¡¡, when he gets home because he's been on Barry's half day grouse, half day pheasant shoot. He'll look like this →

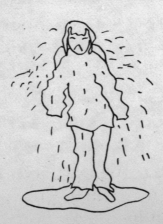

MICHAEL went to the Tennant's the other week with EILEEN, COLIN, STEWART + SANDRA and Sandra's parents, for his first booze-up. (so called). All they did all night was play darts with Colin, Stewart and Pat. [He was what you were like when we were at the Tennant's last, in the same company → BORING] We're sitting here listening to all your Augustus Pablo, Bob Marley records - we've sat on one, scratched two, and dropped two. Its hard to put records on when you're in bed. MICHAEL + STEPHEN have just come back, so we're all sitting here eating

FRUIT CAKE by MRS. YEADON.

Its the next day now - its nice + SUNNY at the moment, although rather WINDY. ALISON + KATIE have just brought CHEZ and

ANDY to the sitting-room door, so we could say "HELLO". We're listening to Stevie Wonder SECRET LIFE OF PLANTS. GEOFFREY has just come in to talk to us. He says you can read deep meaning into whatever colour has been chosen for you.

BRIGIE had a great big slobbery kiss from DENNIS last night, - when he and VAL came. Dennis had raided his supply of heather HONEY which he thought Val didn't know about, to bring some to BRIGIE. VAL announced at the GATHERING that she already knew where it was. DENNIS was most put-out.

SANDRA says the SNOOPY'S are breeding - every time she comes, there are about 3 more.

Some GOOD NEWS- FIONA, of JONTI

+ FIONA has had a little girl
yesterday at 1PM. This is them—▷

😊 👧

MUM has just come in + told us that
the RAF are going to send FLARES
down on LITTON on Guy Fawkes
Night. The BONFIRE has been made
already in EILEEN and COLIN'S
croft.
Anyway, thats all we can think
or now — BORING wasn't it?
So, BYEEE!   love from

Brigid (can't write in bed)
+ Jane (can't write anywhere)
X X X X X X X X X X X
P.S —▷ MUM says keep this
letter!

There was another joint project that week. Brigie had decided that she wanted to organise a few days' holiday for G. and I and she thought of Goathland which we had enjoyed before she became ill. 'I gave Mum a present but I haven't given Geoffrey anything yet,' and she asked Jane to write to our friend Dorle who had recommended the place to stay. She responded with the information and several leaflets, and Jane and Brigie spent a good deal of time debating how it could be managed.

Chris and Alison came again, and she would bring Shez to see her in the afternoon. The horse was there looking through the open sitting-room door at Brigie on the settee when Sister D. arrived. She was shocked to see her patient in a draught, and brusquely dismissed both horse and rider. Brigie was affronted and decided she was 'bossy'. There were some remarks, too, about 'this horror', meaning the settee (she told me afterwards that she and Sister N. had almost decided to 'gang up on us' about this until they realised that Brigie liked it, and thereafter put their minds to helping us adapt) and she had brought a soft sheepskin to relieve the pressure on Brigie's ankles and heels. Already she had her 'polo', the round rubber ring to sit on, and the ankle and elbow bands to save friction on the settee cover. Sister D. insisted, this day, on doing Brigie's hair because she thought it so beautiful, and Brigie began to see her soft side. The doctor came too, and thought Brigie slightly better, but he would come on Saturday evening as well so as to give Mr. N. an up-to-date report on Monday. We knew that Brigie was better than she had been earlier in the week, but there were still the distressing bouts of coughing that she had experienced all through the week, when she would struggle and struggle to release the phlegm and be exhausted afterwards. It was always very upsetting for whoever was there at the time. I would hold her in the way the physiotherapist did in hospital, and long to give a really energetic cough myself to give her some relief. There was a particularly bad one this night, I think, and I can remember Mark sitting there miserably while she struggled.

She had only just got over this when there was a knock at the door. This was one of the very few times when I could not ask a friend to come in: G. was being very upset in the kitchen and Brigie was not fit enough, so there was simply nowhere to take him. I was very sorry as he had travelled quite a long way to see us.

G.M. and Marilyn and Andrew came, giving a welcome boost after the anti-climax of the last few days. Marilyn's secretary had been to Lourdes recently with her son and she had brought back a medallion for Brigie. We thought it the wrong time to offer it to her, but I was touched by the concern of a total stranger. Jane said she would like to wear it for Brigie. G.M. and Marilyn would spend the nights at Kirkby Overblow.

On Friday night, G. said he would sleep in the sitting room with Brigie (after all, he did not snore!). Before she went to sleep, Brigie talked to him and made a memorable statement. She told him how lovely it was now with Jane and Andrew. 'It's all different since I've been ill. It's lovely now with Jane and Andrew and I wouldn't swap that for anything.' Did she know what she was really saying? Looking back, I think she did. She said to me at one stage during this week, 'I love you, Mum, and I love Geoffrey, too.' And to Jane, 'I'm glad we've got Dad as Dad, but I'm glad we've got Geoffrey as step-Dad.' She had never talked about her feelings for any of us until she was ill, and to hear her speak like this was very moving.

She had made similar remarks to Alison about Jane and G. during that week. When Alison talked to me later about it, she told me how much Brigie had changed since she had seen her last. 'She used to talk to me a lot,' she said, 'and she was quite a catty sort of girl really.' Now she found a new sensitivity, and she wrote about what it was like:

Chris and I journeyed up to Yorkshire on hearing the news that Brigie had cancer. At the time I was not apprehensive or really worried because I had a natural optimism about

Brigie. I assumed that things would be all right. However the apprehension came as I knocked on the post-office door. I had never seen anyone ill, still less seriously ill, and perhaps this accounted for my optimism.

At first when we entered I was shocked. The change seemed too terrible and my only thought on seeing Brigie lying on the sofa was how awful it all was. She lay surrounded by furry animals, Snoopies and things and with a clutter of drinks and tissues on a chair next to her. The room was bright and cheerful, which seemed to allay my fears a little. Janet was smiling and normal and even more friendly than usual: it was just Brigie I was scared of. Yet the minute Brigie spoke my fears went, it was as if she had a knowledge of them because she looked at me sharply with bright eyes and said, 'You know you can't be nasty to me now because I'm ill!' This was said as if at last she had won in our lighthearted, bantering friendship and I instantly laughed and felt better. It was as if our positions had been changed and she was the victor and I the defeated.

I sat down and Brigie asked how we were and I said I would like to ride Shez for her. Her face lit up and she said how nice that would be because she had been worried about Shez. Chris and I stayed a long time that day and there were constant coffees and visitors. Sometimes Brigie dozed and as she slept she mumbled, then she would wake up sleepily asking what she had said. As she spoke her eyelids would flutter and she would drift off to sleep again. Everything seemed so peaceful and calm to me that I was happy to be there. When Brigie was awake we talked about her illness and she showed us with a childlike glee and triumph the bandage on her hand where a small lump had been removed. She also showed us her 'polo' (as she called it) which stopped the pressure points on her thighs becoming painful. None of this was done with doleful weariness. Brigie was cheerful and seemed to take an increasing interest in everything. She was not a tiresome, grumbling invalid, quite the reverse. She was bright, lively and excited and she seemed so peaceful and content. Brigie had most definitely changed, and this was to grow more apparent as I saw her more. I think that first day she was very ill, for she was weaker than I would ever see her again but the tremendous thing to me was that she accepted this, not I must add with resignation but with a beautiful, kind and serene acceptance. She was still fighting even with acceptance. Another thing that struck me that first beautiful and terrible day was how pretty she looked with her dark hair on her pillows and her lovely white nightdress and it occurred to me that she was being looked after with a loving and wonderful care. This was contrasted with her accounts of hospital, which she told me she loathed, and as she said this she smiled and looked about her and said, 'But I love it here. Everyone is so kind.'

When I went home that day I must admit I cried partly because of the shock of an illness I had neither been expecting nor prepared for. Yet Brigie's happiness was also imparted to me and so as I became calmer I realised that she did not want pity, she wanted people to share in her experience with happiness . . .

I saw Brigie about four more times and I can only recall snippets of those visits now so I shall not refer to them as individual visits. I took Shez to see her when I rode her and it was lovely to see Brigie's joy at seeing Shez. Once the nurse was there and told me to go away. Afterwards I went to see Brigie and she was angry at the nurse's behaviour, particularly because she had been rude to Janet. Brigie said the nurse had complained about the visitors and how cold the room was and Brigie was annoyed that the nurse had criticised what Brigie saw as good things.

Mark, Katie's half-brother, came with us one occasion to see Brigie, and I remember that Brigie and I teased him about his accent and because we felt he was being pompous about university. She laughed and was quite the old Brigie, the one who would tease and joke about people. Yet there had been a change. She had matured rapidly, become calm, serene and somehow trusting. The change had always been in Brigie, I think, because I liked her for her kindness, yet it was as if one growth had produced a deeper growth of maturity. She had grown exceptionally kind, loving and forgiving. I remember especially how she spoke of Jane and Geoffrey with whom she had had a few problems before. I had remarked on the friendship which had emerged between Jane and Brigie and she said, 'Yes, she has been wonderful and I really love her now. I will tell her so one day.' She also spoke of Geoffrey as having been very good and kind to her and it was this love both from these people and the rest of her family and from herself which seemed to me so incredible. Brigie had both given strength and received it. She had, however, retained her character. She had not become too gentle.

This change gave everyone I saw with her, even friends, the most enormous comfort and strength. It enabled us to enjoy visiting and to come away feeling strengthened by seeing such love, goodness and beauty. Brigie did not want pity or really anything but the presence of her loved ones and to give them something which I shall never forget. Last week as I visited her grave I noticed a bunch of flowers planted there which I think symbolises how I feel about Brigie and that wonderful week with her, a bunch of forget-me-nots.

During the week I had received a long and thoughtful letter from John Robinson in Cambridge. He had heard from Ruth every night by phone: he had been 'thinking and praying so much for you all'. He was coming up this weekend, he said, and:

If you like, I would gladly come and share in a very informal laying-on of hands. As I see it, this is not a piece of magic but an act of identification with a commitment to that power at the heart of things which we ultimately believe is not one of death but of life and love. For the

Christian it is a commitment into the hands of Christ—
and we remember the marks on those hands—to the
power which alone can make any of us whole, whether in
this too rapidly decaying flesh or beyond it. I don't know
what resources of faith and courage and hope Brigid feels
she can honestly make her own, let alone articulate, but
that does not matter. I often think of the healing of the
paralytic in Mark 2, the man who was 'borne of four' and
let down through the roof, of whom we read, 'Jesus seeing
*their* faith said to the paralysed man, "Your sins are forgiven, you are free, get up and walk."' We have no right to
insist, nor I think to encourage people to believe, that the
healing or wholeness shall always make itself apparent
at that level. But I believe faith means being open to
anything . . .

I believed that too, but a service at home could happen only if
Brigie would find it comfortable. I told her again that we
believed that prayers were helping her, that she and all of us
would be put in touch with a power of love and goodness and
that it would strengthen her in her illness. 'No, I don't think
so. I wouldn't like him to come here,' she said. I told Ruth
that we would appreciate a service in the church, though,
and she suggested a laying-on of hands by proxy: the family
could receive this on Brigie's behalf. It would be very good
if other friends and neighbours would come too, I said. We
mentioned it to a few of those around us, stressing that they
should not feel obliged to come, but only if they wanted to.
Ruth and John let others know that it was happening, and
she told me that people were grateful we wanted them: so
many had been very concerned yet had felt helplessly unable
to do anything. G.M. and Marilyn would be there. So would
Michael and Andrew. Stephen would sit with us.

G. got back from visiting his father in Sheffield that Saturday
evening, in time to see the doctor, who talked to the three of
us in the kitchen. He was impressed by the improvement in
Brigie's condition and told us that at the beginning of the

week he had expected her to live just a few more days. He thought she would tolerate the operation and he would tell Mr. N. We were very heartened by his words, all of us, I think, still hoping for a medically inexplicable cure. G. and I had discussed what we meant by the word 'miracle': it meant, we thought, the breaking through of a power of goodness and love which could overcome darkness and pain. We saw the service of the following day as an opportunity for this power to flow into Brigie and into all of us, but at what 'level' the healing would happen, I did not know. It was not right, I felt, to challenge God: surely it had to be 'If it be thy will'. All the same G. said that night, after listening to the doctor, that perhaps Mr. N. would get a surprise when he operated next week.

John had asked me to talk about the service with him. I rang that evening, but was incapable of coherent thought, and all I could offer were three sentences which were running through my mind all the time: 'Be still, and know that I am God,' 'In quietness and in confidence shall be your strength,' and 'The peace of God which passes all understanding . . .' He gave me the references for the readings he proposed: Psalm 139, vv.1–18, 23–4, followed by part of Tillich's meditation which was quoted in *Honest to God*, p. 58; Mark 2 about the paralytic man; and James 5: the elders of the church are called on to be the healing community. At the end, we should come up to the altar rail to receive the laying-on of hands and the congregation would be invited to join him in the sanctuary, as part of the healing community, or to stand behind us, or simply stay quietly in their seats. My only anxiety was that there should be no duress or embarrassment for those who did not usually come to church and he assured me that he would avoid that. G. and I looked up the readings and thought they were very appropriate. We told Brigie what was happening: it was a service to help her and give her strength. I do not think she was worried about it. Rachel and her mother and friends would be here while we were out.

Getting ready for church the next morning I put on the

blouse that Brigie had given me to help me feel that I was taking her with me. As we drove down I explained to Michael and Andrew about the laying-on of hands, and said they should do what was comfortable for them: either come up with us or stay seated. I wondered afterwards whether I should have been more positive about it, but I did not want to put any pressure on them.

We were amazed and touched at the number of people in church. Ruth came over to say that she had prepared places for us at the front, but I thought we were comfortable where we were, in our usual place: G. and I, Jane and Stephen, Andrew and Michael, with G.M. and Marilyn behind us.

We were here, said John, for prayer and healing, in the trust that with man many things are probable, with God all things are possible. He wanted to focus on two differences: that between cure and healing, and that between optimism and hope. Cure was the removal of the physical causes and effects of illness: healing was being made whole in body, soul and spirit. This was not something purely individual: Brigie's family had also discovered a new strength for which they were thankful. 'We are here this morning to draw upon those deeper resources in which all our lives are rooted and joined—to go down, as it were, to the water table, to deep springs too deep for words or tears, to open ourselves to the grace and power in which we live and move and have our being—which as Christians we dimly perceive and confidently trust is a power of love, suffering and triumphant love.' Those words were rich in meaning, and I hoped that many who had come here in extreme urgency would understand about that power: that these were words of the most compelling relevance for Brigie and for us all. Optimism, he said, is based on rosy prospects of which there are not many within us or around: hope, as St. Paul says, is based on endurance and affliction—on resurrection beyond and out the other side of death—on a love of Christ from which *nothing* can separate us in life or in death, in things as they are or things as they shall be.

The service went on, the familiar phrases which had calmed me at times of greatest stress, shared now with all these others: 'in quietness and in confidence shall be your strength . . . underneath are the everlasting arms. Be still then, and know that I am God.' As we knelt in silence I held Brigie in thought, visualising her on her settee, probably by now joking with her friends, and prayed that in spirit she too might be part of this expression of hope and trust. Even more in the next prayer did I try to hold her: 'Open our eyes to thy presence, take us out of ourselves . . . so that in thy light we may see light and in thy will find our peace and freedom.'

Part of Psalm 139 followed, the basis for our belief, we were reminded, that God is inescapable and in all things, including what is most on our minds at this time. The thought here, and in Tillich's meditation,* is concentrated and demanding: 'We are always held and comprehended by something that is greater than we are, that has a claim upon us, and that demands a response from us.'

The second reading related more directly to the theme of healing, that of the paralytic man whose *friends'* faith was the key to what was described as 'the release and unblocking needed at the heart before the power of healing can be let loose within the whole person'. Here was a parallel for us: our faith had brought us together for Brigie. But were we entitled to ask only for her physical recovery? The paralytic man had regained his health through the healing of the whole person: 'Your sins are forgiven you. You are free.' This wholeness of body, mind and spirit was surely what was most needed both for her and for us all, and I felt compelled to pray for that rather than for physical wholeness on its own. In the James passage, there was the call to the whole community: 'Is any sick among you?' he wrote. 'Let him call for the elders of the Church [not simply people with special knowledge or gifts of healing, but the local Christian people as the healing community we are all called to be]. Confess your faults one to

* Quoted in Appendix 1.

another, and pray for one another, that ye may be healed. The effectual fervent prayer of a righteous man availeth much.'

It was time for the preparation of laying-on of hands. We all feel helpless, we were reminded. What can we do? In our own strength very little. But we can open ourselves to the channels of a power greater than ourselves. Then came an invitation to participate in any way that was comfortable: to kneel and pray for Brigie and receive the laying-on of hands with prayer, to take a place in the sanctuary as a member of the Christian fellowship offering the ministry of healing with outstretched hand, to stand behind us, the members of the family, in silent support and intercession, or to remain seated and pray.

I went up first, trying to concentrate on taking Brigie with me in spirit to the altar rail. As we knelt there, it was most moving to hear a great body of people taking their places behind us. I was conscious of a solid strong mass of support, the spiritual support and love symbolised by their actual physical presence literally behind us, and a tremendous unity of deep-felt yearning for Brigie as we prayed for her.

We received the laying-on of hands with the words: 'The healing of Christ, the prince of life.'

O Christ the Master Carpenter who at the last through wood and nails didst purchase man's whole salvation, wield well thy tools within the workshop of our lives that we who come rough-hewn to thy bench may be fashioned to a truer likeness at thy hand.

After the Lord's Prayer we returned to our places. There was the hymn Sun of my Soul, and then the Celtic blessing:

The deep peace of the flowing air to you
The deep peace of the living water to you
The deep peace of the standing hills to you
The deep peace of the Prince of Peace to you.

141

And the peace of God which passes all understanding keep you and her for whom our hearts go out in the knowledge and love of God and of his son, Jesus Christ. And the blessing of God the Father, Son and Holy Spirit be with you always. Amen.

It was over, a profoundly moving service. Everyone came out very quietly, and I wanted to thank people and found, rather embarrassingly, that everyone was kissing me as they came through the porch. I think it was their offering of solidarity to us, but some slipped away with just a smile. It had been a rare gathering of believers and non-believers, and I heard later that Janet Beard had said to John as she left the church, 'I didn't believe a word of it, but I was very glad to be here!' For some it must have taken great courage—for Mrs. Gill, sitting in front of us, and for John Davis who had lost his only child, a daughter, in just this way.

G.M. and Marilyn and Andrew went to the Robinsons', Michael, Jane, G. and I came straight home. We hardly spoke on the way back: it was like coming down from the mountain top. G. helped to bring us back to the plain when we were in our kitchen again (Carol Rawson was washing up yet more coffee cups). There had been one embarrassing moment at the beginning of the service when John announced that we were there to pray for Brigie *Taylor*. I felt G. wince beside me and felt for G.M. just behind us. When we got up G. waited for G.M. as a sign of apology for the mistake in name. The gesture was appreciated. Now, when I referred to the unfortunate slip, G. said, 'I hope they never let him loose at a coronation.' It was just one of the times when his quiet joke would give us a much-needed laugh. He told G.M. later that if it was any consolation he (G.) was often referred to as Mr. Moorhouse.

We went in to Brigie, who was enjoying her friends. She asked me about the service, and as I tried to find words to sum up such an experience she helped with 'Was it moving?' Yes, I said, it was very moving indeed, and that was all that was said. The afternoon was busy with visitors: Eileen and Colin, Val and Kate. G.M. and Marilyn took G. to Skipton for the train and then drove home. Andrew would stay longer. As I had a long overdue shower that late afternoon, and washed my sticky hair, I wondered how we could do the same for Brigie. She hated her hair to get greasy, and it had not been done since she and I did it in the bathroom before she went the last time to Airedale. I planned a method while I was doing my own. Val had already cut her fringe for her on Saturday: now we would get her well supported on her pillows with her head clear of the settee end and we would have a basin on a chair behind her. Jane and Andrew both helped, and we managed, with a good deal of hilarity. Brigie's morale improved with that.

When everyone settled down that night there was time to think about the service. It had been a truly heart-warming experience for us: a coming-together of people from every part of the dale and beyond, all united in their intense care and concern for Brigie and for us. The laying-on of hands meant different things to all of us, I think: for me it was a recommitment to acceptance of whatever was going to happen—I could never simply pray that Brigie would regain her health, although I thought that would be the greatest blessing—and an openness to the strength and power and love that was being offered. I learned in the whole period that suffering and pain have a hidden, positive quality and the service helped to point me in that direction.

# 7

⸺⸺⸺ ❦ ⸺⸺⸺

# *A struggle for words*

*B*rigie hoped that she would not have to return to hospital yet, but after several calls on Monday Mr. N.'s secretary, Elaine, said that he would like to operate the next day, as otherwise it would have to be delayed until Thursday. The ambulance would come about lunch time. How would Brigie feel about it? she asked. I said that she was hoping to stay at home for longer but I was sure that when I explained the circumstances she would accept it. Elaine said that everyone in the ward thought she was 'absolutely marvellous' and that the nurses would be so pleased to hear that she was doing better. Brigie was very pleased when I told her this, and she thought it was just as well to get the hospital bit over, and then she would be home again sooner. She would like Jane to come with us in the ambulance. There was one fortunate circumstance in this timing. Michael was going to Whitby for the week on a geography field course: at least he would not be coming home to an empty house again until Friday. I remember asking him before he went if he wanted me to let him know 'any news' about Brigie while he was away, and he said No. I mentally agreed with him: it was best to keep his two worlds separate, and if there was anything to hear he had best be at home. I rang G. to ask if Andrew could take the car to Bradford for us: he would come about 4 p.m.

Brian, with Glen this time, pulled up, and there were lots

of jokes and good humour. We set off, but had not gone far before Brigie felt sick. The jokes stopped immediately and they pulled in, and all care was given to her. It was the hazelnut yoghourt that she had before she left, she decided. There were no more jokes until Brigie felt better and went to sleep. I knew that everyone would realise who was in the ambulance as we went down the dale and Mary Miller waved from her garden, unable to see us wave back through the dark-tinted windows—Brian told us some tricks they had played with those. We stopped in Skipton for Brian to go to the bank, and he was nearly knocked out, he said, by a painter on his scaffolding. Brigie was able to lift herself up and see the cause of his near accident.

Jane went up to the ward with Brigie when we got there, and I registered her downstairs. On the way up I met Brian and Glen. They were different people now that I was alone, full of concern for her and her next operation. They complained that they were never told anything about their patients, were not allowed into the wards to collect them, and so were left in ignorance about where they felt pain. This made the work of settling them comfortably so much more difficult. They assured me of every assistance when Brigie returned home, and that I could have a lift to the hospital with them.

Brigie was right at the bottom of the ward, and Jane had arranged Pete and the bears on the window-sill. Flowers from G. were waiting for her and more from G.M. arrived later. We were all trying to be cheerful, and Andrew's arrival with a bunch of carnations helped to break the long afternoon. Brigie was dismayed when he took off his donkey jacket and uncovered his only available T-shirt, the elderly one with all the acid holes in it, and she thought with a roll of her eyes that he had better keep his jacket on after all. They took out the stitches in her hand, and she held on hard to Jane with the other one. We stayed till the end of visiting, promising to be there as early as possible in the morning, stopping for fish and chips, I think, on the way home. We were all hoping that

Brigie's improvement meant that the cancer was regressing: such things had happened before. When I spoke to G. that night and told him Mr. N. was convinced that the Rythmodan tablets had regulated her heart-beat and produced the improvement he said again that he thought Mr. N. might be surprised when he operated.

Andrew was going back to Bangor on Tuesday. We would go to the hospital to be with Brigie till her operation and then he would get the train from Bradford. We found her very low in spirits and she had not slept very well. She kept saying, 'I'm really glad you're here.' It was a long wait for her injection, as another operation had taken longer than expected. When Andrew was out for a few minutes, she looked at me very miserably and tears came into her eyes.

'Why do I feel so bad today? Is it just because I'm back in hospital?' I said I was sure it was, but already she had got some of the time in hospital behind her, and the day for coming home was getting nearer. She wept about two tears, and then asked if anyone would see she'd been crying. I assured her they wouldn't, and there was a rustle of porters to take her to the theatre. She had been right about not crying again after she knew she had cancer; those two tears were the only ones.

Andrew and I went to the station and had some coffee. I had to leave soon as I was going back to Litton to collect Jane and wanted to be in the ward again when Brigie woke up. I had about an hour at home, and we set off with the sandwiches that Jane had made.

Brigie was just momentarily awake when we arrived and there were new furry creatures on her locker, the two chipmunks. G.M. had been in, having driven up from Broxbourne. 'They're gorgeous, Dad,' Brigie said when he returned in a few minutes. She was now back at the top of the ward, having oxygen again, and she had a tube in her back draining the lung into a jar under her bed. I saw Mr. N. and he said there was a mass of tumour which he had not been able to touch, but he thought he had relieved her breathing and stopped the accumulation of fluid. He had obviously not experienced the surprise that G. had hoped for. G.M. had talked to him about the operation too. 'Was it, in fact, to stop her from drowning?' he asked the doctor. 'That's right,' said Mr. N. 'It was.' We stayed till the end of the visiting hour, and Brigie looked as if she would be sleeping that night, at least. G.M. came back to Litton with us. Jane went in first and came rushing out to me—'Mum, the fairies have been.' There was another massive carton from Margaret, a large joint of cooked pork with apple sauce, flans, cakes, pies. How kind and how welcome. I simply did not feel like cooking and after a long day at the hospital nothing could have been more relished than the flan and the coleslaw that we found in our kitchen.

On Wednesday G.M. and Jane went early to the hospital. I would look after the post office and take the shop order into Skipton on the way to Bradford.

I think Ruth came up here that morning: I was still worried about talking to Brigie about dying. We talked about the dreams she'd had and how she thought she saw Pompah sitting in the chair. Perhaps there was an unconscious aware-ness there, Ruth suggested, but it had not yet reached the conscious level. I must try to get in touch with that buried knowledge. I was worried that she was not voicing her real thoughts because she did not want to give us pain. I wanted to find some way of indicating to her that I, for one, was able to bear the information. I prayed about this, and asked Fairacres to do so too. Until I had talked to her about it, I could not speak to anyone else, although to one or two close friends I think I indicated that it was a good deal worse than we had thought earlier. It must be getting obvious that we had stopped talking about treatment, and that the operation was purely palliative.

I got to the hospital in the early afternoon, when it was nearly time to go to the station and meet G. G.M. offered to go down as I had been there only a short time. G. remembers Brigie being very sleepy that afternoon but, as the effects of the anaesthetic wore off, her eyes became very large and brown and she would smile with them, and just sometimes with her whole face. At other times, she slept peacefully and we watched those short breaths, noticeably lifting just one side of her chest. It was difficutlt to demonstrate our affection: she was too sore to be hugged and one hand was immobilised with a drip. One could just kiss her and hold her other hand, taking care not to disturb the tube draining into the jar. When she tried to talk she had trouble with her words, not being able to find the right one and giggling at her confusion. I thought it was still the effect of the anaesthetic but Jane had doubts. She dreamed a lot and made unintelligible comments, but once she said something about 'waking up in the morning with a coal miner'. G.M. laughed and said he thought she could do better than that, and she smiled. At times she was very much aware, the only one of us who noticed that Jane had cut her own hair that day. Mr. N. was saying that he hoped to get her home by the weekend and that was very good news for Brigie and all of us. He told me how rare these cancers are, so unusual that there is some disagreement among specialists about what to call them. He did, however, give G.M. a name: it was rhabdomyosarcoma. A doctor would probably see only about one or two cases in a lifetime's work. Brigie's slides would go to a central collection in London as this was the only way they could build up a body of knowledge about them. If Brigie's condition had been recognised when the 'ganglion' appeared they would have amputated her hand, if not her arm, and then given her blunderbuss chemotherapy, and three months later, probably, another lump would have appeared somewhere else. It gave me a horrifying picture of what last summer might have been like: at least Brigie had been spared the trauma of mutilation and distressing treatment, all most probably for nothing. As it was she had a very good summer, and I was grateful for that. Mr. N. said he would have her back at any time if we could not cope, but we said we very much wanted her to stay at home. He met Marilyn's father that week and told him he thought she would be better at home with us.

When we were not with Brigie we were pacing again those endless B.R.I. corridors. It was too cold to go outside for a cigarette now, but Jane had found a basement corridor with a bench and an ashtray, and there we would take the chance to talk to each other and often to have a quick cry. There was one young porter who would smile and ask me how she was. But one could not stay there long, as Brigie might be asking for us, and we would go back to the seat outside the ward and, as Jane described later, 'stare blankly at the radiator' on the other wall. The days seemed endless and yet we would not have been anywhere else in the world. The inactivity of it, coupled with the strain, was exhausting, and we decided to repeat the pattern of *that* day's visiting: G.M. and Jane to go early, and I would go later and stay longer. That meant six hours rather than ten at the hospital. It would also give me some time to catch up at home: it was difficult to keep things going on the practical level, even though Val and Ruth, whenever they looked after the post office, also did a large pile of ironing.

I felt guilty, however, when I got there on Thursday in the early afternoon. Jane said Brigie had been very low in spirits and kept asking why I was taking so long to get there. I sat with her a long time and gave her all my attention. She still gave me no opening for honest talk, and when Jane came to give me a break I met Mr. N. at the entrance to the ward and had a long and helpful talk with him. He told me how upset he was about Brigie. When he had her on the operating table, he said, he realised how thin and wasted she was. 'She's got big boobs and thighs, and that's deceiving, but when I cut through the muscle layer there's nothing there. I can operate on all these old people [and he gestured to the ward] and I can operate on small babies—all right, it's very hard for a family to lose a baby—but this age . . . I've got daughters of my own about this age. Our society is just not geared to teenagers dying: teenagers don't die.' I told him about my worry and my doubts about his colleague's advice that dying should not be talked about. That was where he disagreed with him, he said: they were of a different generation and now most doctors believed in honesty. I told him about her dreams, especially the one where Dr. Y. had come, saying that she should go back to hospital and then die. Perhaps you could say to that, he suggested, 'No child of mine will die in hospital.' The indirect way, using the third person, and associating the other members of the family, would disperse the harshness of the information. It was so difficult, I said, to be honest without depressing her.

'That's the really awful tightrope and you've got to walk it. I've got the easy part, I'm just the technician, but you've got to do the caring.' I was very impressed with his involvement and his sensitivity, and was to use his advice later.

When I went to move the car he was just ahead of me, slumping along weary after a day's operating.

'You must be tired,' I said.

The mood had changed.

'I've got to get out and buy some fireworks. My daughter doesn't give a damn about all this bloody surgery. If I don't get some fireworks, I'm a failure as a Dad.'

I felt a great admiration for that human and skilful doctor.

I went back to sit with *my* daughter. The others had gone back to Litton. Now recovered from the anaesthetic, she had been moved to the far section of the ward where there were no other patients. She was sleeping quite a lot as it got dark outside, and through the window behind her I could see the shooting rockets and hear the bangers down the hill in Bradford. I dared not think of all the other bonfire nights that we had known—I must not cry—and I hoped that she would remain unaware of what night it was. She woke, though, after one loud bang, and I told her it was the fire-works. She was only mildly interested. When she was awake I stroked her arm in the way she liked. She had told me about this game that she and Michael played, taking turns in running their fingers up and down the other's forearm, but I was not sure that I got the movement right. (When I told Michael about this after she died, he said with refreshing openness that he always did it for her but she could never be bothered to do it for him.) She was peaceful and looked as if she was settling into sleep when I left. I gave her a kiss and said I would be back as soon as I could in the morning. I had decided that I would come early the next day, and give her a surprise. It was the last day in hospital for her, and I would stay right through. It was a question of pacing oneself out and knowing how far one could go: husbanding the resources.

I drove back through the fireworks and saw the remains of Litton's bonfire next door to us in Colin's croft. I hoped to get in unnoticed, as that jolly occasion was beyond me, and I succeeded. The atmosphere inside the house was difficult: tension and the close proximity of us all was beginning to tell. I was surprised that it had not done so earlier. G. apologised for it later: it was his fault, he said. We had a meal and went to bed. I, for one, was grateful for oblivion.

I left early the next morning with G.M. to go to the hospital. G. and Jane would come over in the afternoon, after the weekly ceremonial of balancing the post-office accounts, and G.M. would go to Leeds to meet Marilyn. They would go back to Kirkby Overblow. Mr. N. told us he thought she could go home the next day. We sat with her all morning, either one of us or both, and in the early afternoon Mr. N. came to tell her definitely about going home. They had a bantering conversation. Why couldn't she go home today? she asked. She was much better and perfectly ready to go.

'Look here. You had major surgery three days ago. Do you want to get me prosecuted for negligence?'

'But I'm much better. Why can't I go?' Here was the old challenging Brigie reasserting herself. It was no good, though: she could not persuade him.

It was quiet in the ward after that and Brigie was dozing. G.M. was sitting beside her and I was slightly behind him (as the bed was by the partition only one side of it was available). The staff nurse came round with the drugs trolley and stopped at the bottom of the bed, explaining to Brigie that hers were not ready yet: as she was going home her chart had gone downstairs to the pharmacy so that they could get her pills ready. And then Brigie asked her shattering question: 'Are those the pills for when I'm dying?'

The three of us were dumb for a few seconds, and then we all said something like 'No, the pills for taking home with you.' G.M. gave me an amazed look over his shoulder and the staff nurse moved on. I cannot remember what was said then, but I knew I wanted time to think. Was this a question that came straight out of her subconscious mind without her realising what she was saying (how do I know what I think till I hear what I say?) or was she taking the opportunity of telling her parents that she knew? Over a year later I am still not sure of the answer, but I think it was the latter.

At the time I was still thinking of my conversation with Ruth about subconscious awareness, and I decided to tackle it from an angle. I wished afterwards that I had gone straight in, and asked her why she had said it, but at that time it seemed too bald. After G.M. left to go to Leeds I asked her instead about a dream she had about Pompah.

'Did I dream about him? I don't really think about him now.'

I said I was interested to know whether he looked the same as we knew him, or whether he was different 'now that he is dead'. It was a clumsy way of introducing that word: she could not remember and the conversation did not lead anywhere.

She was quiet again for a while and then she suddenly made, for me, one of her most moving statements.

'I love you so much, Mum. You're an absolutely lovely Mum.'

I was so overcome that I could only put my head on her shoulder and cry and tell her how much I loved her too. She could not have that for too long, though, and helped me to recover by giggling and saying, 'Oh, for goodness' sake, don't cry on this one!' (her new nightie). I was still damp-eyed when G. and Jane came in a few minutes later and had to get away and restore myself.

We all talked about how it would be the next day. Val's mother had lent a bed-rest to support her pillows. 'And the fire will be on,' said Brigie. She knew we loved her, all sitting round her bed making happy plans for her homecoming. She had just one more night in hospital. Jane and I would get a lift in the ambulance to Bradford. We left her in good spirits, but I cried much of the way back, thinking of what she had said to me. I was so caught up with this that I did not tell Jane and G. of her question about dying until we were back in the house. I remember G. standing there, half-crying, half-awed, saying, 'How can a sixteen year old accept that she's dying?'

There was no time then to absorb all the implications of what she had said. Michael would have returned from his week's field course in Whitby to an empty house yet again. Eileen had filled that gap as she had so many others. He was full of his experiences when he came in and I was glad that he had had a break from the tension, but, sadly, the evening was busy and we did not have time to hear all that he had to tell us. Andrew arrived with his student friend Dave, who had given him a lift from Bangor. He stopped for a meal with us and then left saying that he would collect Andrew on Sunday evening.

Looking back on that day, I wondered if Brigie had sensed a cloud waiting for her, and made a point of saying two important things while she was still in control.

# 8

---⁂---

# *November 8th–14th*

$T$he drive that Jane and I had in the ambulance to Bradford next morning proved more eventful than we expected. First there was a stop at Brian's house to pick up his wife's milk: they had recently had twins who were in hospital, and the supply had to be delivered every day. We were waved off by his wife and other two children, a lively household obviously, particularly at night, Brian remarked wryly. I enjoyed talking quietly to him and was glad Jane could cope with Glen's jokes, for which I was not in the mood. There was some clowning about at Airedale with the milk, but Brian got it safely to its destination and we were on the way again. We talked about the twins, and then he said, 'You all seem to be coping remarkably well. Some families that we see are in absolute mayhem.' He told me about a friend of his who had had lung cancer: his wife had not been able to continue nursing him at home when his breathing became too distressing. This was my worry, I confessed. We very much wanted to keep Brigie at home: might we need oxygen? Yes, he said, 'and we would always bring it up for you'. They would bring anything we needed, they assured us. I discovered later that the Grassington chemist knew all about us, and he, too, was prepared to bring drugs to us, a total journey of twenty miles. It was very reassuring to know we had this support.

As we got near the hospital, messages started coming through the radio and they both suddenly became tense and professional. The blue light started flashing as they were the nearest vehicle to the accident: they tore into the forecourt, we leapt out, and they were off. We went up to the ward: there was a quick greeting to Brigie and we hurriedly packed her things and the flowers. There was no physiotherapist giving her exercises this time. A porter arrived with the trolley and he and a nurse lifted her on, none too gently, and it hurt. She and Jane set off, and I stayed to have a word with Mr. N. He told me again that this was the worst sort of experience for him. 'She's so bonny. You might have her with you for a family Christmas,' he said, 'but you might not. I'm just so sorry that the doctors are so helpless, that's all.' I told him he had helped us very much. He was very affected and said he thought we were an extraordinary family 'to be taking that kid home like this'. I managed to say that it was very important to us, shake his hand, and go quickly as I was in tears by then. I always cried when people were kind.

The trek to the ambulance stand gave me time to recover and Brigie was already installed. She had to be higher, though, and Brian and Glen propped her up, but she kept sliding down. She had been put on the trolley the wrong way round, and they would have to turn her.

'We won't hurt you, pet,' and they were very careful. It emphasised their point that it would be better for them to go to the ward and get it right in the first place. Brigie was comfortable now and could look out the back window as we went along. We heard all about the accident they had just been to, and then she slept for some of the time. She woke just before Lane End and could pick out landmarks as we came up the dale: her eyes shone.

All was ready at home—family, flowers and fire, and she found the bed-rest comfortable. Brian and Glen had coffee and then left: 'Now don't forget—anything you need.' Brigie had parcels to unpack—more furry animals, and they took their places with the others along the settee back. Even opening parcels was too much for her: her fingers did not have the strength. This homecoming was much more subdued than the last. She was feeling very poorly. Sometimes we talked quietly so as not to disturb her, and at others just sat there silently. It became important to concentrate on the moment, to try and get Brigie to have something to eat—she wanted potato soup yet again but ate hardly any—and to see that she was not getting overtired. People came and went, but there was usually someone sitting on the settee or the pink stool, holding her hand.

The bedpan was not so easy now, as Brigie could not lift herself up, and Jane and I found it hard to manoeuvre her on the settee. Sister D. had brought her own little pink commode the week before, but Brigie did not want to use it then. However, it became essential now. Later the nurse told Jane the story of this little wickerwork cabinet. It had been given to her by Sister Bunnett, the old and respected nurse who had worked in Kettlewell for years and whom she had nursed. Sister D. knew that one day there would be 'a special patient' who would have it.

During the afternoon Marilyn told me what Brigie had just said to G.M. She had been sleeping, and as she woke she said, 'It was great!' He asked her what had been 'great'. 'We were all praising,' she answered. I was amazed and awed at her use of a word which one would have thought so alien to her.

I got out the mattress that evening and settled down in the sleeping bag. It was some time during the night that I saw Brigie behaving oddly. She had her leg and eiderdown right up the side of the settee and was pushing all the animals over the back, looking at them in a very hostile way. She did not respond when I asked her about it, and did not seem to focus on me at all. I thought the new painkillers might be making her confused. In the morning, though, she seemed as alert as ever, and got ready to see Helen, on her way home from Sheffield. G. took Helen in and talked quietly to Brigie:

Helen spoke later about her father's gentleness and rapport with Brigie.

Andrew had gone up the hill to fetch Shez: he wanted to bring her down for Brigie to see. Jane and I were determined to get her out to the door when they came: walking was very difficult for her now (Mr. N. had told me he thought she had permanent nerve damage in her left leg). It was important that she should see Shez before Sister D. arrived: we remembered the previous time and still thought of her as the 'bossy nurse' who would put a stop to such unconventional proceedings. G.M., Marilyn and Andrew arrived with the horse and we got Brigie into her dressing gown and over to the open door where Shez was. There was so much joy and love in Brigie's voice as she said 'Oh hello, baby,' and patted Shez's neck. 'Hello baby, you lovely baby.' She was with her for a few moments. I found it unbearably poignant, and cried silently as I supported Brigie from behind. Jane, on the other side of her, saw my collapse and kept control. We got an exhausted Brigie back to the settee and I retired without having to speak. Jane managed the gentle encouraging talk that was needed.

Later that afternoon, when Helen was saying goodbye to Brigie she told her to look after herself. 'If I can't look after myself,' Brigie said, 'Mum or somebody else will.' After she had gone, Maurice rang to say he would call either before or after evensong at Arncliffe. He talked to G. and me for a while and then said he would like to see Brigie; he wanted to say a prayer with her. I was doubtful how she would feel about it, and asked if I might consult her. 'Just say I'd like to give her a blessing, Janet.' Brigie was slightly surprised but said, 'Yes, all right.' We all went in and Maurice spoke to her for a very few moments, very naturally and in a matter-of-fact way: he was very glad to see her again, he said, and he wanted to give her a blessing to help her. He knelt and put his hand on her head and Jane noticed that she closed her eyes. He just said, 'The peace of God which passes all understanding keep your heart and mind in the knowledge and love of God and of His Son, Jesus Christ; and the blessing of God the Father, Son and Holy Spirit be with you to help you and strengthen you. Amen.' There was a moment's silence, and then he got up.

'Thank you,' she said, looking up at him, 'that was lovely.'

He would come again on Tuesday, he said. 'Goodbye,' and he gave a smile to her and everyone in the room and we came out.

'That child is at peace,' he said to us. 'I could tell from the way she accepted the blessing. I know she's at peace.' After about two minutes he was gone. A short visit, but an important one. Brigie had not just been polite to him. After we had gone, she said to Jane, 'That was really nice, wasn't it?' He came every two days after that, with always the blessing and the smile, a short chat with whoever was about, Jane or Andrew or Michael, an easy unforced joke perhaps, and then he was gone. If anyone wanted to talk, he would stay. That service to us must have been very costly in time and petrol— it entailed a very long drive—and we appreciated it very much.

Dave called for Andrew that evening and they went back to Bangor. G.M. and Marilyn went home.

Brigie was still having trouble with her words. She would try out several sounds and still not get the sense she intended. She would giggle about her muddle at first, and we had to laugh out loud sometimes because some of her newly coined words were hilarious. Once when she was feeling specially close to Jane she said, 'But we can't get married, because we're twisters.'

Our laughing often irritated her, though, and we felt very guilty about it: that was the cause of one of Jane's 'collapses', as we called them, after being at the hospital one night. She had upset Brigie with her giggles at the wrong words, but I knew that these lapses were relatively unimportant. Brigie was secure in our basic love and concern, and that underlying fact was the important one. She got very cross and frustrated when she could not make us understand, and I was worried about this confusion, caused, I thought, by the painkillers. It threatened to cut off communication and there were important things to be talked about. At times, too, she had bad dreams. She would wake and look around with a terrified expression, and she seemed to see strange appearances round the room even when she was awake. When I asked her about her dreams, she said some were super, but others were 'horrible'. Once when she woke up, she asked accusingly, 'Why are we moving?'

I said we were not moving: *I* didn't want to. Did she?

'No, of course not. I love it here. I really love it here.'

On Monday morning G. drove to the station and went to London, leaving the car at Skipton. Ruth came and we sat with Brigie for a while. She told me that people had been very glad to come to the service the previous week, and some had asked if they could not go on helping in this way regularly. She had offered to take a short service of prayer on Wednesday afternoon. Jane and I would be glad to go if we could. We talked about the problem of Brigie's confusion and I decided to ask the doctor if we could change the painkillers. It was Dr. K. who came later and he said he thought she had cerebral secondaries and that her confusion was caused by fluid on the brain. It was time to start diamorphine, he thought. I was very reluctant: we still hoped, in spite of the medical evidence, that she might recover, and we did not want her hooked on heroin. I knew, too, that the drug, while giving relief, also hastened deterioration. He said there was another drug as well which would help to control the fluid temporarily, and this might give her a few days of lucidity. I asked him if I might speak to Mr. N. about it as G. and G.M. would need to be convinced that diamorphine was absolutely necessary.

I tried to call him that afternoon at the hospital, but he had gone home. The staff nurse was very reassuring about diamorphine: they had patients on it, and they were able to get about normally. It would be a mild dose. If I still wanted Mr. N., though, I should ring him at home. I did, and his wife knew about us, and she said he would ring when he got back.

This was rather different from the formality of approach to most consultants and I was very grateful for it. He rang soon after: he did not doubt that Dr. K. was right. This was what he had hoped would not happen so soon after the operation. He said the painkillers would not make her confused and he approved of the drug to control the fluid. We should start diamorphine. I gave her the first dose that night and she said it was horrible, 'quite alcoholic', but she had a much better night afterwards.

On Tuesday Kate was to ride Shez to Conistone: she would stay in the stables there. It was pouring with rain, but she rode Shez past the window, and Brigie was able to wave. She seemed even more confused and frustrated and I saw a fresh difficulty if her friends from school came. She still looked lovely, but she was very ill and weak and this, combined with the confusion, suggested to us that the time for visitors was past. I rang Miss Kent and asked her to tell the girls of this development; that she was not well enough to see anyone. It came as a great shock to them all: they had not realised that her illness would go at this terrifying speed. The girls saw Miss Kent in a new light that day: she was very upset herself at having to tell them this news, and they could see the depth of her feeling. She told me later that she had to send Joanne home because she was so heartbroken. She offered to come herself with Brigie's certificates if that would be any help. It was a kind suggestion and I said I would let her know later. I had many letters in the next day or two, from her teachers and from friends' mothers: the underlying message of them all was that they wished they had come earlier, but they had not realised the time was so short. Nor had we, so it had been impossible to warn them. I had even hoped that when she recovered from the operation I would be able to take her in a wheelchair down to the farm again, at least, and perhaps to see Shez.

The confusion became even more upsetting that day. I felt quite helpless when I could not understand what she wanted and it was often Jane who was more in tune with her, and could interpret. Sometimes we would try two or three possibilities in answer to a request and still be wrong, and Brigie would give up trying to make us understand with either a resigned look or with silent fury. This must have been a heartbreaking isolation for her: we simply could not make contact.

This frustration reached its climax that night after we had settled, she and I, to sleep. At least I thought we had settled: I was desperate for sleep after several broken nights. But Brigie could not get comfortable and I couldn't understand what she was saying. I tried sitting her up on the settee with her feet on the floor to give her a change of position, but that was not right and she lay down again. We changed positions several times and we tried the commode. She started giving me extremely hostile looks and saying 'Mum!' in tones of freezing fury. Then from her sitting position, she leaned down and got hold of my sleeping bag, indicating she wanted to sleep on the mattress. Before I could cajole her any more she suddenly flopped and got her legs into the bag. There was nothing I could do but try to prop her up with all the pillows, but I knew it would be bad for her breathing. It could not be for long, but I lay down on her settee, longing for sleep. Five minutes later we were up again. By now, my patience was running out, and when she got back to the settee I let fly. Anger might be effective where long suffering was not.

'Now look here, Brigie, I know you're ill, and I'm very sorry. But I've got to have some sleep tonight so that I can look after you tomorrow. So let's stop all this messing about and settle down!' It seemed to clear the air and we slept. I still had many chances, though, that night to remember how hostile she had been to me, and I had to come to terms with it. There must be a more positive reaction than simply being hurt. After a good long think, I realised that it must be a release of her feelings of anger and frustration, and I should feel privileged that she was secure enough to offer them to me. My part was to accept them and absorb them. She had, after all, given me the extremes of her feeling: I had been joyful with the love and should not feel differently now with the anger and the hate. Somehow I must show her that I could bear it, and that it did not make any difference to my feelings for her.

Dr. K. came the next morning and thought she was poorly, but hoped that the new drug would give her a respite. I told him about our worry about the diamorphine's addictive properties. That would not happen, he said. If a drug was taken as medicine it would not lead to addiction: the motive was the key factor. At some stage that morning Brigie said to me, 'I was horrid to you last night, wasn't I?' I said I knew she was angry about being ill, that if I could help by letting her be angry with me I was pleased, and that I loved her very much. We were calm after that.

Ruth was taking the short service for Brigie and G. might get back from London in time to go. I wanted to go, too, but the nurse was late. Would Jane go on her own? She said she did not think she could manage that and we both stayed. G. arrived afterwards. It had been very moving, he said, and Ruth had given him her notes which I could read later. Brigie was very glad to see G.: he usually got some of her best smiles, and he was very good at sitting quiet and relaxed with her.

We thought we were approaching the last stage of her illness. Gladys and Dick, we decided, must be given the chance to come and say goodbye to Brigie. G. rang them and they arranged to come on Friday with Lucy, Brigie's god-mother. Brigie was very weak, and that was two days ahead. I hoped they would not be too late. We explained that they should spend just ten minutes each with her as she was so ill.

In the early evening I took Ruth's notes and went to sit with Brigie while I read them. Jane followed me in. G. had said to her, 'She will need her glasses: it will make her cry.' (I often used my glasses to hide damp eyes.) He was right. The prayer that Ruth had said that afternoon in church on my behalf was a profound expression of what I knew, as yet in theory only, to be the positive way.

I pictured our friends kneeling in the choir-stalls as I read

Ruth's words. 'We come together holding Brigie in our hearts to draw water from the well of life that we may give each other to drink.' There was an echo of the idea that she and I had talked about together.

So let us first make ourselves empty of everything that is taking up space. We let go our frets and worries, our anxieties and petty occupations, the jobs we are in the middle of—everything that is cluttering us up, emptied away.

O Lord of life, scour me and cleanse me that I may be empty and bright in thy light, waiting to be filled.

Christ who is amongst us and between us, fill us with your loving strength and pour into us your everlasting life that we may be able to nourish and sustain each other. We hold Brigie between us in the power of this love, sustaining her by our prayerfulness and trust in life or death.

There was a reading about the nobleman who came to Christ asking help for his son, and then another prayer.

Grant, O Lord, that Brigie may have fullness of life and wholeness of body, mind and spirit. A whole life for a whole person is our prayer for her. If it is possible let her be restored to us in this life. We do not ask this as a sign and wonder but because we love her with a yearning human love and would have her with us. But if love demands, we ask that she may know another life where our prayers can be fully answered.

And now we hold the family in our prayers, giving thanks with them for the miracle of love and joy that has come to them and through them to us through Brigie, enriching all our lives, remembering them each in turn—Michael, Jane, Andrew, Geoffrey Moorhouse, Geoffrey, and a special prayer spoken on Jan's behalf:

Dear Lord of Life. I have carried this child within me. Through the pain of my body and the cutting of the cord between us, I gave her life in this world. If it must be that she and I must share another birth through the pain of her body and the grief of my soul, give me the grace to let her go lovingly and joyfully, that she may know a fuller life yet live for ever in my heart. Amen.

Janet, go thy way, thy child liveth.

And finally it is Brigie's turn to speak. Waking from a dream the other night she said, 'It was great! We were all praising!' Let us make this a reality for her.

[She read part of Psalm 138] I will give thanks unto thee, O Lord, with my whole heart . . . and praise thy name, because of thy loving kindness and truth . . .

Let everything that hath breath praise the Lord.


The service ended with St. Paul's triumphant assertion, 'For I am persuaded . . .' and then the grace.

I could cry silently, the light was dim and Brigie was half-asleep, so my state went unnoticed, but as Jane read she sobbed. Brigie suddenly woke up, and remembering former irritations, she asked sharply, 'Is she laughing again?'

That prayer had made us open and ready, and I found myself saying, 'No, Brigie, she's crying, and I'm crying too. We're crying because you're so ill, and we're sad.' There were a few moments of silence and then more words came. 'We're sad, but we're not unhappy—there's a big difference—we're happy for you because you're going to be very happy.'

Jane said, 'You don't need to worry, Brigie. You'll be all right.' Brigie drifted off to sleep again. For me, a great burden was lifted: we had said something real in an abstract way and Brigie was peaceful. This was the first of three short, important conversations on consecutive nights.

The next morning Brigie was very weak and sinking. She could take only small sips of drink, and the nurse was not bothering her with washing. She was awake hardly at all. Really close friends must be given the chance to say goodbye. G. went to ask Eileen and Colin, and she came that morning.

Brigie was hardly aware, but she sat with her for a few moments and gave her a kiss. Colin came later when I was asleep upstairs. That strong man was terribly shaken. Margaret Dagett rang. She had heard about Miss Kent's talk to the girls and was very upset. She said it would help her boys a great deal if they could come for just a few moments. They would come on Saturday. I made phone calls: Mrs. Hartley would bring Janet and Abigail on Friday and Pat would bring Joanne on Saturday. I had to explain to everyone that it was just a matter of coming in and giving Brigie a kiss: it was unlikely that she would know them. It was very hard for all her friends, and I wanted them to see that she was peaceful and comfortable.

Even so, she could still surprise us with her sudden awareness at times. She remarked on something I was wearing one day, and said, 'Yesterday she was a brown Mum.' And, looking at me again, 'You need a new pair of trousers. We'll have to see what Father Christmas can do,' and her secret, conspiratorial smile appeared. She was able, that morning, to see the flowers from R.A.F. Dave, but we did not read her the full message on the card. 'Your helicopter will be arriving on November 19th,' it said. Mark and Kate were still coming every evening and one of them would sit holding her hand. We came to feel that this was a privilege, and we had to make sure that everybody got a reasonable 'turn'. Kate could not let herself believe that Brigie was dying: she would try to rouse her with snippets of news and be overjoyed when conversation was going on in the room and Brigie would suddenly join in when we thought she was asleep.

'She doesn't miss a thing,' Kate kept saying. Mark was very quiet with Brigie: he would just sit looking at her, grieving, but even so we realised later that the full knowledge had not reached him either, although we had told them both.

Sometimes people's rejection of the facts was troublesome: we would know that Brigie had had enough of a particular visit, especially if people were simply discussing their own affairs, but it was difficult to move them without hurting feelings. I would be inwardly screaming, 'Don't you realise that Brigie is dying?' as they sat on, not taking any particular notice of her, and there would be pain in her eyes. I was worried that Michael was not getting enough time with her: if there was someone else in the room he would simply go upstairs. I kept saying, 'Brigie's time is very short now,' but I do not think they believed me.

After these, too-casual visits, Brigie would say, 'That was awful.' She was very sharp about people: 'I don't think I like her very much,' or even 'I can't stand that woman' (accompanied by a rude sign). Her perceptions were very acute, picking out artificiality or sentimentality, and she could not tolerate pity. She liked people to be themselves. When Steve came in one night, loud and jovial with his 'Hello, blossom! Do you know me?', 'Of course I do,' she said, delighted.

On Thursday evening I was sitting with her again. She had been half-asleep, but she suddenly roused and focused intently on the end of the settee and said very definitely, 'I've got to go soon. He's waiting for me. I've got to go!' She was trying to lift herself on her pillows.

I was very anxious that her grandparents would see her the next day and this made me say, 'I don't think you need to hurry. You can take your own time. I'm sure he'll wait for you.'

She looked at me, and there was a sad and anxious expression in her eyes. 'But you can't come,' she said.

'No, not yet. But I'll be coming later, and then I'll see you when I come.'

'Did I know you?' she asked. She was still getting muddled with her words and I was sure she meant 'will' rather than 'did', so I answered, 'Yes, we'll all know each other later when we come.'

She went to sleep again almost immediately.

There were going to be many short visits on Friday, and everyone was going to find it very difficult. For some of them, we felt sure, Brigie would perhaps be aware and know them, if even for a few moments. But it was totally a matter of chance, impossible to guarantee. She would perhaps go through the whole day without knowing anybody. I think Stewart and Robert came in the morning, and before lunch Gladys, Dick and Lucy arrived. His diary recorded the visit:

> . . . to Skipton where we stopped for Gladys to buy a dozen roses for Brigid. We arrived at Litton at eleven ten and we were greeted by Jan and Geoffrey, and Jane gave us a cup of coffee. We spent a quarter of an hour each with Brigid. She is very pallid and has much trouble talking, yet when I was with her, she knew me, called me Grandad and asked me to kiss her—how pitiable to see her—this almost voluptuous child now in the last stages of cancer-death and accepting the inevitability of it! She knows her end and is accepting it beautifully (if that is the right adverb).

The next day he wrote: 'Although I seemed to sleep well, Brigid's lovely face has been haunting me—if death is as beautiful as she makes it, why ought we to fear it?'

They were all very upset when they were here: I tried to tell them that she was prepared for death and very peaceful, and this, I felt, was because of all the support of prayer that we had. Dick asked me how we managed to feed her when she was so ill. When I told him that she had eaten very little for several weeks, he had to go and look out of the window for rather a long time. It was so hard for people to accept the reality of it all.

Dr. K. was disappointed that the other drug tried, dexamethasone, had not relieved her confusion. It was about this time that I asked him if he could remember when it was that Brigie had first gone to him with her 'ganglion'. He looked up at me in horror, and I realised that up to this point, he had not realised that this was the primary cancer. He had a great shock. Her card showed that it had been on July 2nd. Mr. N., he told me, had said that the bio-life of these cancers was about five months from first symptoms until death. Brigie had already had longer.

Later in the afternoon, she seemed to revive and wanted to sit up on the settee with her legs down. We were always glad when she was ready to do this, as the nurses said a change of position was good for her. Jane sat beside her with Brigie's head cradled on her arms: she was very adept at making Brigie comfortable like this. They were still there when Mary Ann came. G. had rung her at the gift shop to say that Brigie was sinking and she had dropped everything. She did not expect to see Brigie sitting up like this, and even less did she expect Brigie's reply to her 'How are you?'

Brigie said, 'I think I'm dying, but I'm not quite sure.'

As Jane said afterwards, it was more than difficult to reply to such a statement, and Mary Ann was very shaky when she came out. Brigie was still aware when Janet and Abigail came for a few minutes after school. They told her about a new pup and she wanted to know what they were calling it. For those of us who were with her all the time, her capacity to switch, as it were, from one world to another in the space of a few minutes was quite breathtaking.

G.M. and Marilyn came that evening, laden with food again for the next few days. Marilyn seemed to spend most of her evenings in Broxbourne cooking for the weekend in Litton. They always came not only with dishes ready to be put in the oven but with other material benefits, notably alcohol, which we seemed to get through in great quantities. There must have been something about our metabolism at this time which allowed us to consume without any effect except relaxation. It was not only us, because everyone who came seemed to need a drink, and G. became so embarrassed by the number of bottles that accumulated that he declined the facilities of the council rubbish van, preferring to take them surreptitiously to the Settle tip. This time, G.M. and Marilyn were going to stay the week, as we thought Brigie could not possibly live more than a day or two longer. Andrew came home as well and he, too, would stay. He simply could not concentrate down in Bangor, and his tutor thought he should be here. We were very glad. G.M. and Marilyn would spend their days here but sleep at Kirkby Overblow.

When everyone had settled down that night I was sitting with Brigie. Again she had been asleep, but woke up and just said, 'I'm going to die soon, Mum.'

I tried to say that she would be happy, would always be looked after, and that she would not be lonely. She made a small, impatient gesture with her hand as much as to say (as she would have in the old days) Don't go on about it—*I know*. You don't need to worry about me, you know!

I was silent: I had been clumsy again. She went back to sleep at once.

On Saturday afternoon Joanne came with her parents, and Gayna with her mother. Brigie was hardly aware, but knew them for an instant or two, I think. Nigel and Michael were coming at night. Margaret rang to say they were desperately anxious to do something for us and could they bring some logs? She guessed that we had a fire on day and night. It was a very thoughtful offer. Brigie was able to greet them, I think, and they stayed just a short time. When I came into the kitchen I found another horn of plenty from their mother. I was so overcome with the kindness of it that I burst into tears: they seemed to cope with my collapse. The kitchen was full of large bodies drinking G.'s elderberry wine and describing their own efforts. The logs had already been put in the garage. Kate and Mark were still seeing Brigie every night and Val came in most mornings, and so we felt that all the people who were important to her had been given the chance to say goodbye.

I began making other specific plans for when she died. I told Sister N. that it was very important for me to do everything for Brigie myself. I was not going to hand her over to undertakers. She told me all she could, and left a package of equipment. Sister D. gave me a list of telephone numbers, including her own. I was to ring her first, when Brigie died, even before the doctor, and she would come. We talked to

Maurice about burial at Arncliffe and decided on Raymond Harker at Kettlewell as the undertaker. We were expecting the end at any time.

I had just received another letter from Mother Jane at Fairacres. It came on a large card with a clear and colourful picture of a butterfly, wings outspread and perfect. When she had answered my first call for help, she had told me that one of their sisters, Elvira, was dying of cancer, 'very bravely and cheerfully'. I did not want, at that stage, to link Elvira and Brigie together because I so much wanted Brigie to live. Now I felt differently.

> My dear Jan [Mother Jane wrote], Our Sister Elvira is very near *her* end now, and I said to her that she's like a butterfly emerging from the chrysalis of her poor diseased body. Now, after showing her this, and telling her today's news of Brigie, I'll send it on to you because I believe it's saying something true, even tho' there's no human comfort, I fear. You must try to believe that all the rich potential of her life *won't* be wasted, but 'renewed, transfigured in another pattern' as Eliot puts it . . . We are all very much round all of you in love and prayer, my dear—Jane SLG.

I thought about Sister Elvira a very great deal, the brave and loving nun dying at the same time as Brigie. It became very important to me that she should die first, and be there to help Brigie. I could not wish for a more loving companion than one of those marvellous women. I remember sitting up with Brigie one night and writing rather emotionally to Mother Jane, wondering if I dared to hope that Elvira might be able to hold Brigie's hand in spirit. It was not logical, of course; if one believes in a fuller life beyond death it should not matter about the detail of who is there, but for me it seemed a very reassuring link between this world and the next. I did not hear again until after Brigie's funeral.

It was becoming more difficult to keep Brigie comfortable on her pillows. She would slide down until her head was at an awkward angle and too low for her breathing. She no longer had the strength to lift on her hands as we righted her. Sister N. devised a way for three of us to lift her together—one behind the settee and one in front, hands holding wrists under her legs and back, and someone behind to support her head. We managed very well, but it meant that I had sometimes to get Jane and G. or Andrew up in the night to help. Sometimes if she was sitting with her legs on the floor we could swivel her round single-handed into the right position and we got quite good at this from the commode. As she got more and more sleepy, though, we could not always get her there in time, and then the nightie and the sheepskin would have to be changed. She hated being disturbed in this way: she simply could not be bothered with the commotion, however gently and quickly we did it, and would become fretful and impatient like a child. Imperceptibly, we started encouraging and per-suading her in terms appropriate for a little girl. This fitted her own feelings, I think: she began calling me 'Mummy'. Jane would say, 'You're a good girl, Brigie.' It was at these times, too, that she started saying she wanted 'to go home'. At first we thought she was just muddled and believed she was still in hospital, and assured her she was here, with us. It came to seem much more than that, though, as if she saw some bright and inviting place ahead of her, and was im-patient to get there.

'Geoffrey, Geoffrey, help me to go home,' she would say as he sat holding her hand. 'I want to go home.' And once she woke up and said with great urgency, 'Come on, come on—push us, push us' as if 'they' were in a boat waiting to go across water. At other times, when we could not understand what she wanted, she would be angry and her eyes would flash. 'This is the limit,' she said once. 'If it goes on like this, I'm going home!' Then we would have to try not to laugh, or at least not let her see us laughing.

I realised afterwards that for us the borderline between laughter and tears was very thin, and both provided a relief from tension. Marilyn has remarked that there was laughter all through that time, even when Brigie had gone beyond it; and it is strange, thinking back now, to imagine how we could possibly have laughed while Brigie was dying, and yet, apart from one or two instances when we were ashamed, it all seemed entirely appropriate. There were different kinds of laughter: the quiet, relieved smile and chuckle at G.'s throwaway humour or Brigie's remark to the ambulance men, the rueful laughing at oneself struggling to recover from a quick cry, grateful for the good fortune of living in a shop with its unlimited supply of tissues, and the shaming, uncontrollable giggles that beset Jane and me once or twice, and which we wince to think of now. We were getting more and more tired, and we were vulnerable to those sudden, incongruous happenings that could set us off, uncontrollably giggle-prone as we have always been. Normal life had to go on, even though something so abnormal was happening, and we went on being ourselves with all our weaknesses. I wish I could remember some of the quiet, warm jokes that G. made so effortlessly, never sharp or intrusive, often self-deprecatory and always very funny. That humour was very much in keeping with the atmosphere.

That was certainly quiet and peaceful. Someone was always with her: it was Jane who had first said, 'I don't think we should leave her alone at all now.' Often it was her sitting there holding Brigie's hand, smiling when she woke up, ready to give her a Wet One that G.M. had brought, if she was hot, or a drink of blackcurrant or lemonade through the flexible straws that Val had thought of. Just that intense concentration on her, even when she was asleep, was tiring, and Jane would be there by the hour. Not many of us could do that for such long periods. For an active, outdoor person like Michael it was difficult, and hard for me, too, during the day when I would always remember something that should have been done, or some call that should have been made. My time was at night: I had given up trying to lie down as there were so many calls, and as the tiredness accumulated it was harder to get out of the warm sleeping bag quickly enough. I would sit in a chair beside her, dozing when she was asleep, instantly alert again when she stirred, staying more alert than ever between 2 a.m. and 3 a.m. because that was when I believed she was likely to die. We had Andrew, now, to help with the watching and he became much involved. He studied the best position for her pillows, and helped to lift her when she slipped too low. There were other services for her too: he got some baby oil one day, and rubbed her feet with this very gently and carefully. Their roughness had been bothering her.

So it was at the end of her first week at home. It was just the family now, with Mark and Kate, drawn closely around her, and close to each other, more aware of each other's difficulties than we had been before, and trying to keep everything right for Brigie. I think the atmosphere was good—other people said so—and certainly it seemed calm and peaceful. 'What a marvellous, peaceful scene,' Janet said when she came for about two minutes one evening, bearing more of her ample tea cakes, 'the cats by the fire, the flowers, and Brigie sleeping on her settee.'

# 9

~◇~

# *November 15th–21st*

With Andrew home we developed a pattern of watching which meant we all got enough sleep to keep us going. I would go to bed at about 10 p.m. or 11p.m., either before or after G.M. and Marilyn went back to Kirkby Overblow, and sleep for a couple of hours. At about 1 a.m. I would take over from G. or Andrew and stay with Brigie until about 7 a.m. when I would wake Jane or Andrew. One of them would be on call, too, during the night if I needed to move Brigie. I would go to bed until the doctor or the nurse came.

Those nights with Brigie were very quiet. She would sleep most of the time until restlessness would indicate she was ready for more diamorphine; I sat beside her, dozing or thinking, sometimes writing a short letter or two, keeping the fire going, very attentive around 2 a.m. to 3 a.m., giving her a drink from time to time and making tea myself. All through those long nights I knew that we were being supported, and it was a great reassurance to think of all the people who were praying for us. I was usually in a half-awake zombie-like state, and my own thoughts and prayers were disjointed and staccato. I was leaning very heavily on other people's and my own were very specific: for Brigie's peace of mind, for sweet dreams to help her on her way, and for the small group of us so closely involved.

We all had our different times and ways of being quiet or

withdrawing. G.M. had brought up his canvas needle this week and he spent a lot of time in the barn stitching Shez's rug which had got badly torn on the barbed wire when she was unattended. There must have been a lot of grieving during those cold hours up there thinking about his daughter slipping away, but he would emerge to sit with her again, to clear out the fire, or to wash the endless piles of coffee cups that accumulated. For G. too there was grief and anxiety; he had been through this kind of experience before with Joan. He would have to go back to London on Tuesday, but on Monday night he suddenly announced that he was going to see Maurice. He did not talk about it that night, but later he told me that he felt that even at this stage something might be done to save Brigie's life and he had to talk to Maurice about it. He came back and tried to encourage Brigie to have some tomato soup. It was a panicky time for him.

Brigie was very weak indeed. She had no strength even to lift her hand: when she raised it to touch her face, it just dropped down again heavily, and it was about this time that she took off her bangle and her watch. She had already taken off all her rings, except for Mark's signet ring, and given them to Jane. In return Jane had given her the Lourdes medallion which she had been wearing for her, but now the watch and bangle were removed too. It seemed almost as though she was divesting herself ready for death. Earthly adornments and pleasures, one felt, were now left behind. That assumption, however, would have been wrong. She was asleep one night, and uttering unintelligible comments in her dreamy state, but quite suddenly her expression changed: her lips moved in a really erotic smile and she said, quite clearly and definitely, 'I want to fuck.' The words and the expression passed in an instant, leaving me feeling very shaken. I had no idea then whether they applied to real or imaginary experiences, but we know now that there had been the former, fairly soon after we came to live in Litton.

That was the only such allusion: her sister and brothers were the important ones now. The bond with Jane was very strong. Brigie would sit upright on the settee sometimes with her head on Jane's shoulder, the strong sister cherishing the poor thin weak one. They were a very poignant sight: one all yearning love and deep concern, the other frail and failing, but trusting. Once I went in when they were holding hands and Brigie looked at me with pain in her eyes and said, 'Mum, we can't get married.' She had talked to Jane about being together always, 'but', she said, 'you've got to live here and I've got to live there.'

One evening Jane had been with Brigie for some time when she came out to me and said that I should go in. There had been a marvellous conversation with Brigie who had been using remarkable words. She had talked about 'the leaving of the soul' and 'the grand and the glory', and then she had been singing, and it sounded like a hymn. 'You should go in, Mum. She's in a really good mood.'

All expectation I went, and found just the opposite. She looked at me with hostility. To everything I said she responded with eyes thrown up in extreme irritation. When I did not understand what she wanted she made her remark about this being the limit and threatened to 'go home'. Jane looked rueful and I tried more conciliation, but it was no good. She looked at me with fury and said, 'Do you want to go now?' so it seemed best to accept my dismissal. It hurt, of course, but I had to giggle about the way she had put me in my place.

I had to accept, as calmly as possible, that there were times when she did not want me. Jane was her most favoured companion and I sometimes felt apologetic for intruding, and yet guilty at the same time for not being there. There was no time or energy to fret about whether I was failing her: I had to go on looking after her, indicating that this rejection did not alter my feelings for her, and finally stoically deciding that there were times when she would have to put up with me anyway.

Sometimes at night all four would be together, and they gave her a lot of strength. G. had to come out one night because it was so moving. 'It's a lovely sight in there,' he said, almost in tears, 'Jane and Andrew and Michael just sitting there around the settee looking at Brigie. There's no anguish, it's quite calm: they're just there with her, and it's absolutely lovely.'

She was aware that many friends, some far distant, were with her in thought. She had many letters—a large bundle collected by Joanne from all her friends at school had come some time ago, and Kate had read these to her. She was still getting a special postcard from Granny and Grandad every day, and now letters came from friends of former times. Emma and Ellen, from Broxbourne days, wrote her long and newsy letters, and Elaine from Sheredes. Some older friends, I realised, had great difficulty knowing what to say to a dying sixteen year old. I spoke to G.'s John in Sweden one night and he asked me what would help. I was able to tell him that Brigie had talked of Mark and Robin recently, remembering the summer at Westhill Road and, she had said, rather sadly, 'I expect they've forgotten me now.' John's response to this was a letter which gave her much pleasure.

Dear Brigid [he wrote], Just a few lines to say that we are all thinking of you. Mark and Robin . . . talk a lot about you since it was often you who changed their nappies and generally looked after them when we came to stay. Mark especially I know is very fond of you. Robin is too young to remember when you looked after him that summer three years ago but he remembers the time last year when we went to look at your horse. I wish we could all come and give you a hug but it's not easy with the North Sea between us. I am sure you will know that with this letter come our warmest thoughts of you and our fondest love . . .

It was letters like that, expressing love and care, and remembering past connections, that gave her happiness. Her Skipton friends were writing frequently, and so were Alison, Rebecca, and other neighbours from Westhill Road, old friends from the stables at Broxbourne, and children were sending her pictures they had drawn. Local children brought them in on their way home from school, Katie Beard painted Shez for her, and David and Nathanael, her young cousins, sent their colourful offerings from America. Kate, now seven, wrote a letter with drawings. 'Dear Bridgie,' it said, 'I will come to see you son. I can canter now and I will come with you to see your horse and I will bring a picture of a horse. I am not very good on hores. Love Bridgie from Kate.' A friend from the school bus sent her a huge Snoopy card of his own making. 'Get well soon, Brigid,' it said, 'coz—we miss you.' Our friends and family were writing to her, too, and sending presents—every day more heart-warming proof of how many people were thinking about her and caring so deeply. We would spread the reading of the messages through the day, choosing times when she was aware enough to understand. A cheque for five pounds came from the Littondale Charity. Jane went into Skipton one day with Stephen and bought her another furry animal, a gold coloured lion. Practical help was still coming to us, too. One night Eileen sent over an enormous meal with all her varied side dishes: there was so much that it fed us for about three days. Jean Dolan had made us pies and would bake our Christmas cake, and Janet our Christmas pudding.

Even this week, with Brigie so weak, there were unexpected visitors. R.A.F. Dave, in the area for an exercise week, came on Monday morning. I was asleep, but I heard how shaken he was to see her so low. And then on Tuesday Val told me that Kate had met David and Martin, the Stainforth lads, on Saturday night and told them about Brigie. David had cried; they wanted to come on Tuesday evening. This would be very important to Brigie if she was conscious enough to recognise him. I had thought the attraction was, perhaps, one sided as he had not seen Brigie since Kilnsey Show, but Kate had not told them up to now that it was serious because it might upset Mark. (I hoped they would not come together.) I was slightly nervous about meeting them: my only contact before this had been a cheeky greeting after Brigie had disentangled herself from an embrace in Stainforth. As I drove off with the girls a voice had said, 'Hello, Mother,' in tones which had not endeared me to the speaker. They poured into our tiny kitchen with Kate, and though they were quiet and slightly awkward, I could see they had a natural confidence and a sense of humour capable of adapting to new places and people. It was an easy meeting and I took them in to Brigie. I had not told her they were coming for fear of disappointment, and though she had been asleep she roused and recognised David with a delighted smile. I left them for about half an hour; it was a very important visit for her and they should have longer than the others. They came out very quiet and subdued: it had been a shock for them. Kate made them some coffee, and then they went, asking if they might come on Friday. Martin would ask again to borrow the Land-Rover. Nobody thought that Brigie could possibly live much longer: she had been taking only sips of liquid for several days now and sometimes, following Gladys's suggestion, I would soak a tissue and put it on her lips for her to suck. It was easier for her to manage than actual drinking. Marilyn was not coming the next day: she had made the helpful suggestion that she stay at her mother's and do some cooking. We were getting very congested and there was little space or time to cook here, and tired, tense bodies, all six or seven of them, need hot and tasty food. I remember I asked G.M. that Tuesday evening before they left if he wanted me to let him know in the night if Brigie died. I stayed very alert that night, but Brigie slept peacefully. On Wednesday she was still very weak, asleep most of the time. She was obviously dreaming a lot: smiling in her sleep and murmuring unintelligibly. We longed to know what was going on in her mind. I wanted to give her the hugs that had helped before, but she was too frail and it would pull the long line of stitches down her back. Once when I made this wish aloud, 'to show you I love you', she murmured, 'a big hug to show my endearance'. Some of these new words she made were lovely, and some, even now, funny, and I wish I could remember more of them.

It was another peaceful night, and when I left her with Jane and Andrew in the morning I hoped she would not die while I was asleep.

When I came down later that Thursday morning, it was quite different. We could hardly believe it when Brigie woke up, alert and bright, and asked for a drink. She would like a cup of coffee, she said, and my hands shook as I made it. She drank it all and enjoyed it. At intervals during the morning she had considerable amounts of the chocolate drink (Carnation Build-up) that G. had bought for her. During that day, she must have taken about two pints of fluid. Sister N. was amazed at the difference when she came, and we talked guardedly about 'the strange things that can happen'. 'One is entitled to hope,' she said, 'but not to expect.' I dared not allow myself to get euphoric, but it was marvellous to have Brigie talking coherently. She put her watch and bangle on again. G.M. and Marilyn came in with all the cooking she had done and they were overjoyed. Eileen came, and Jack left off his round for a few minutes to come and see her too. When G. came back that evening the full group, hopeful and happy again, was complete. Her sleep that night was of quite a different quality and I, too, slept much more.

The next morning Marilyn presented her with a bottle of Dubonnet, her favourite drink, and she celebrated her better state with a drink then and there. Eyes were shining all round as we toasted her. Marilyn had talked to her sister who had nursed terminal cancer patients, and she had said that anyone taking as much fluid as Brigie had the day before was not about to die. We were agog to hear what the doctor would say, and were disappointed that it was not to be Dr. K. that day. His colleague was coming to Litton for a shoot and he would come here in place of Dr. K., but would not, we knew, be able to appreciate the contrast. He arrived at lunch time looking very rural. As G. said, 'I thought it was the doctor but he looked like the vet.' Sister D., however, was amazed at the difference, quite delighted, and decided to give Brigie a

180

full wash. She was able to lift herself up again, the first time for over a week.

When I was asleep that afternoon R.A.F. Dave came. He had been passing the house all week, he said, wanting to come in, but too depressed after his visit on Monday. Now, seeing her so different, he started to talk very positively about the future, somewhat to G.'s alarm. He would go riding with Brigie, he said, up the Stainforth track, and the helicopter would be coming in January to give her a ride. I think it was this day, when I came down and told Brigie I had been having a sleep. 'Oh,' she said, 'you were tired. You look lovely now,' and she touched my face in sympathy. David, Martin and Kate came again in the evening, and were delighted about Brigie. They stayed with her for about an hour, and she was tired but happy afterwards. Kate told me later that Brigie had been very lively: she had asked David to put his arm round her and give her a kiss. Then, seeing the bandage on his wrist, she had asked in distaste, 'What's that?'

'Orf—I got it from the sheep.'

'Ugh,' she said, 'you'd better go away. I might catch it.'

Before she went to sleep that night, Brigie put out her hand and took mine, and said she wanted to talk about the future. Which future, I asked, for us all or just hers? 'No, my future,' she said.

Did she want to talk about it now or tomorrow?

'I want to talk about it now.'

'What are you thinking about the future?'

'Well, there's someone who went away to college to do A levels . . .'

I realised she was thinking about Alison, and I said, 'Yes, you can either do A levels at school or you can go to a college.' She might feel that she wanted to do this when she was better. It was something to be considered and we would discuss it. That was all, and then she went to sleep. We had another good night.

Brigie woke up very bright again on Saturday morning. Andrew was with her and we were in the kitchen when he

181

suddenly called 'Mum!' with great urgency. We rushed in, feeling that something dreadful had happened, to find him supporting Brigie, who was standing up. She had asked him to help her up, and when she was on her own feet suddenly announced that she was going into the kitchen. There was no gainsaying Brigie when she was in a mood like this. I got a chair and cushion, and Jane and Andrew lifted her on this, a difficult manoeuvre past all the shop boxes in the passage. She sat in the kitchen for a few minutes, looking round with great pleasure, and we were delighted to see her there again. The return journey was better organised: Andrew went backwards with the chair and Brigie put her arms round Jane's neck to steady her. They were both bent over very awkwardly, but the happiness on Brigie's face was richly rewarding. G. was beaming with pleasure and G.M. and Marilyn were delighted to hear when they arrived.

This was a big day for Michael, too—Lads' Day on the grouse moor, the first for four years. He had been talking about it for weeks. He set off full of spirits into a very damp morning: the mist got thicker and we expected them back early. By about 3 p.m. the fog was well down on the hills. G.M. and Andrew were with Brigie and Marilyn, Jane and I were in the kitchen when the phone rang. It was Stephen, saying that Michael was lost on the moor and he had come back for his motorbike. He was checking that Michael had not come home another way before he went back to rejoin the search. It was very nasty news: the fog was very thick and Michael had been missing for three hours. However, as we reasoned together, with about twelve gamekeepers up there on the moor they, if anyone, should be able to find him. Fortunately for us we had only about twenty minutes' suspense. The phone rang again: it was Michael ringing from Starbotton and G.M. and G. went round by car to collect him. Stewart, I think, took the message up to the moor. Michael, separated from the others on a drive, had twice found himself in the wrong dale: the second time he had given up and gone to the nearest house in Starbotton. After he had made his phone call the lady asked him how 'that girl in Litton is getting on'. When he told her that she was his sister, she said, 'We're all thinking about her over here.' He came back wet and jovial, and told Brigie all about his experiences. His friends Bruce and Pete had some ribald comments to make to him that night. They were making a notice to pin on him, they said: 'If lost, return to Litton P.O.' Dennis, we discovered, had been so worried that he had forgotten to eat his dinner.

Later that afternoon Brigie said she wanted to get dressed. With great excitement Jane and I sorted through the heaps of clothes that had not been worn for weeks and painfully slowly got her into jeans and blouse. The effort did not give her or us the happiness we had expected: the clothes showed up her pitiable thinness, and she looked down at her baggy jeans with distaste and disappointment. Nor was she comfortable with the constriction, and we got her undressed again fairly soon. When she was lying down, though, I reminded myself that the hollows at the sides of her eyes were much less sunken than they had been a few days ago: already the nourishing drinks had begun to fill out that dismaying gauntness. She could sometimes regard her thinness as an interesting phenomenon. When Michael and Nigel were here that evening Jane came out to tell us of Brigie's latest trick. 'Guess what she's doing now!' Jane said, spluttering with mirth. 'She's got her legs right up in the air showing them how thin they are!' We all enjoyed this further indication that Brigie was still being very much herself.

We had another celebratory drink that evening, Brigie with her Dubonnet, and then G.M. and Marilyn went back to Kirkby Overblow. After everyone else had gone to bed G. and I were with her and she suddenly became very agitated about some problem that we could not fully understand. She was sitting upright on the settee: she wanted, she said, 'a beedle . . . or . . . a wheedle, or a seedle'. It must surely be sewing that was on her mind, so I said that it would be better to wait till the morning so that we could sort it out then. G.

183

sat down beside her and put his arm round her—he too could make her comfortable like this—and he explained very gently and quietly and in great detail what he did when he had a problem late at night, how he always decided that it was not a good time to tackle difficulties, and how he always felt able to deal with the task in the morning when he felt better after a good night's sleep. She listened very intently, and gradually became calm again. They sat there very quietly for some time. Then Brigie looked around at the fire and the picture that Jane had drawn of their bedroom and put up on the wall for her to see, and she said, 'Why is this room so lovely?' I said I thought it was because we were all here together, thinking as I spoke of the three sleeping upstairs and G.M. and Marilyn who had been here so much. There was not much more talking and then she went back to bed and settled down for the night.

# 10

November 22nd–December 1st

G.M. and Marilyn were here in the morning and would set off for Broxbourne after lunch. G. was working at home. Marilyn remembers that one or two girls came to see Brigie that morning and she seemed to feel a strong compulsion to tell them all about her illness from the beginning. It was a great effort for her against tiredness but she completed it step by step, and when they had gone she said, 'God, I'm glad that's over.'

It was a quiet afternoon, and Jane and Andrew were with Brigie. I think she even felt like hearing some of her records again, and when Margaret Walker rang to ask me to go round for a cup of coffee I felt I could be away for a short time. I thought she was asking me just to give me a change of scene, and it was refreshing to be outside again, the first time in two weeks. In fact she had something to tell me, she said, and she was very hesitant about starting. She explained that she was normally very sceptical and this was not the sort of thing that she would naturally take much notice of. But it had come her way, and she had to tell me.

About a week ago she had been preparing her parcels and happened upon an item in the *Yorkshire Post*. It was about a Liverpool healer, and according to the text he had had considerable success. She hesitated, but felt she had to get in touch with him about Brigie. Last Wednesday night she had rung the number and explained her concern. Brigie would be connected by thought, she was assured, from the moment she had made the call and they would post more information for her to pass on to us. Margaret said it was late on Wednesday night, and she described the odd sensation at that time. She sat in her kitchen for about two hours, feeling very strange, as if her mind was buzzing with energy, unable to get up or do anything. As the next day or two passed she heard about Brigie being suddenly better and she wondered. The promised packet of information had come on Saturday but she had no time to read it immediately. The thing that she found hardest to tell me was that therapy for absent patients involved looking at this man's photograph at certain specified times. Some friends of hers came in soon afterwards, and I left feeling very confused. One thing I was very impressed with, though, was Margaret's concern which led her to make the enquiry, and with her courage in telling me about it. She is both sensitive and practical, and her matter-of-fact approach to problems made her the last person to be carried away by quackery. The effort she had made, against her own grain as it were, compelled me to consider what was in the package.

I was just starting to tell Jane about this when Maurice arrived to give Brigie her blessing. His coming at that moment was a great blessing to me: I needed help in thinking this out. The mere act of telling him made it easier to sort out my own questions. We had given God the chance, as it were, to heal Brigie, and now what were we to make of this new experience? By taking notice of this healer, were we just thrashing about? (God had failed us, let's try somebody else?) It was impossible for me to think clearly about it. Maurice was very good. He could understand, he said, if I wanted to try anything or anyone. Certain people, he believed, did have a gift of healing and God works in mysterious ways. Who knows but that he works through a healer, such as this, and as this had come my way it was right to try. He was very calming and reassuring. He went in and gave Brigie a blessing as usual and left us all feeling better.

G., Andrew, Jane and I read the leaflets. G. said that one could not dismiss a thing like this. He had always believed that if Brigie were to be cured it would be by metaphysical means. So at 7 p.m. I settled down to show Brigie the photograph, feeling slightly foolish, I must admit. I told her that this was a picture of a good man who had been able to help people who were ill, and that he was thinking about her now and trying to help her. She looked at the picture and said, 'He looks . . . like . . . Michael . . . ?'

'Parkinson,' I suggested, and said that I thought he resembled him too. That was all.

Other things had to be attended to. Brigie announced that she would like to sleep upstairs. The manoeuvre had to be planned in detail. She sat in an armchair while we transferred bed-rest, sheepskin and pillows, and then Jane and Andrew carried her on a chair to the bottom of the stairs. We could not see how they could lift her on the chair up the stairs, and so very slowly and painfully they helped her up, but she had a lot of trouble with her leg. It was a great triumph to get her into her own bed again, and I prepared to sleep in Jane's. When G. came in to say good night and asked Brigie what it was like to be back in her own room again, she said, 'It's absolutely gorgeous!' Before we went to sleep I thought I should try showing her the photograph at 11 p.m. I got it out and started on the explanation, but she said, a bit impatiently, 'You showed me that before.' I left it at that, wondering if such a cursory glance could have any possible effect, and thought that in the strange logic of the thing it probably could. It was not a good night, however. She had a lot of pain in her leg which the diamorphine did not cope with, and I snored. Once I remember waking to hear this desperate voice saying, 'Please, please!' She told Dr. K. about her exploit the next day and said she was not going to try *that* again.

How could we explain this sudden improvement in Brigie's condition? All along, I had tried to keep an open mind. I knew it was possible that there could be a breakthrough of power and goodness, and that Brigie could experience what some would call a 'miracle' cure. I had prayed that if it were possible, this might happen, but I had never felt entitled to a total faith that this would be so. That seemed to be throwing down a challenge to the Almighty, trying to force his hand to do what we wanted. There were high moments, though, during those few days when I believed that a breakthrough was happening, and perhaps the healer in Liverpool was an agent. Was the sudden improvement on Thursday a result of Margaret's phone call? Brigie's new energy and her determination to use it in activity was perhaps the beginning of a new phase of recovery. Her friends in Skipton, I was told later, had their own explanation, and it was the romantic one: she started to get better when her long absent boyfriend came to see her. Other explanations would emerge later.

I was still allowing myself a muted hope on Monday morning, even though Brigie seemed less alert. I told myself and the others that this could be tiredness after the colossal effort of going upstairs. Jane and Andrew got her down again, and we decided to put her on the other end of the settee to ease pressure on her leg, which was still painful after the strain of walking. Andrew took G. into Skipton to catch the train for London and then went shopping to buy Brigie more of her favourite 'Tramp' soap that Helen and Moira had sent from Edinburgh. She was absolutely thrilled with this. 'Oh, Andrew, that's lovely. Come here and let me give you a kiss!'

Ruth came that morning and we talked about the healer and other healers she had known. She was as open-minded about it as Maurice. I was still feeling that Brigie might be winning when Dr. K. came, and we were in high anticipation about what he would find. He joined Ruth and me in the kitchen after seeing Brigie and he did not disappoint us. It was incredible, he said. For the first time, he had heard breathing sounds from her right lung and her liver was reduced in size. Not a lot, but significantly. Could this be a remission? Ruth asked. He explained that it could not, as remissions were achieved by means of treatment, and Brigie was having no treatment. What then, Ruth asked, was the medical explanation? He said he had hoped that no one would ask that question. There was no medical explanation. I listened with mounting excitement, and then he asked me what I thought was an amazing question from a doctor. 'What do you think has caused this improvement?' I was not feeling either courageous or articulate, and sensing that he was a sceptical scientist I just said that metaphysical factors might be the answer. Somewhat impatiently he replied that he was looking for practical causes. Fortunately Ruth was able to expand my feeble opening, and pointed out that we felt prayer was a highly practical activity, that there was a level of healing which was beyond the purely scientific and medical one, and possibly we were in touch with it. He remained unconvinced.

In spite of the improvement that the doctor had found, we all knew, that Monday, that Brigie was less well than she had been the previous four days, but we did not admit it openly. She was drinking less and sleeping much more. She was so sleepy that it was impossible to get her to focus on the photograph, and it was obviously going to irritate her if I tried. I decided to ring the healer and ask advice. I got through eventually and started what I thought would be quite a long and detailed conversation. It lasted, in fact, about three minutes. There was a very down-to-earth Liverpudlian voice saying, 'Hullo, luv,' and when I explained Brigie's very sleepy state, he simply said, 'That's all right, luv . . . Just put your hands on the sore parts. That's all you need to do.' At these particular times? I asked. 'Any time at all—we're all linked up in the subconscious anyway.'

He obviously had no more to say, so I thanked him and rang off. It was rather an anti-climax. I took his advice, though, when she was asleep, and put my hands from time to time over her right lung, her hand and her leg. Sometimes she felt the pressure and brushed me aside, and sometimes I stayed there for a few minutes, trying to concentrate my thoughts on a power which might help, a mixture of prayer and relaxation that no doubt did me good, even if it did not reach her. I was still slightly embarrassed by the procedure but if there was a chance that it would help Brigie it had to be done.

I wrote to Miss Kent at this time, telling her that it seemed right to have some of the girls to see Brigie again, if only briefly. I wanted her to know about the improvement in Brigie's condition, and I said I did not rule out the possibility of non-medical reasons, but that we were trying not to be too euphoric about it and I was not going to voice this hope to the girls.

On Tuesday morning I went to bed as usual when Jane and Andrew took over. I always felt very bleary when I emerged, and that morning I remember feeling especially lifeless. Jane and Andrew were subdued and silent too: we all knew, although we did not yet acknowledge it in words, that Brigie was sinking again. It could no longer be explained as tiredness from the weekend efforts. Practical activity was a useful antidote and gave us a change of focus. The room had become very messy and Jane and I gave it a good clean: the result improved morale. Brigie watched our efforts and said she wished she could help us.

While I worked I thought about my conflict within. Was I, her mother, failing Brigie in not having total faith in her physical recovery? Was G. right in his earlier feeling that if only we tried hard enough and believed firmly enough in the seemingly impossible, we could be the agents of her recovery? The burden of all my fragmentary prayers was for Brigie's inner wellbeing, and asking for physical healing always carried the proviso 'if it be possible'. Up to now, it had seemed right to follow the rhythm of how she was feeling; to be positive and hopeful when she was feeling better and wanting to talk about her future, and to be equally positive and trusting when we talked, albeit obliquely, about dying. If instead I had refused all along to accept the possibility of her death, could I have changed the course of events? Even now, should I try to think myself into such an attitude? Was her life slipping away because I lacked faith?

These questions had to be faced, especially now when the hope of the last few days seemed to be lost. The inward debate went on. The reasons for being unassertive still seemed right: how could one throw down a challenge to God and expect an affirmative answer? Would this not be a kind of spiritual blackmail? And would not an attempt to *will* Brigie to live put a possibly distressing pressure on her and make her feel a failure if she could not respond? Surely it was better to follow her natural rhythm and help her to accept death calmly and trustingly as she had been doing? But the doubts remained.

Very fortunately Maurice was coming that day, again just when I badly needed to talk to him. He had spoken earlier about the parents' will being very important and I knew he would give good guidance. I explained my worry. Was I wrong to have given up expecting a miracle?

'But the miracle has already happened, Janet!' I did not stop to ask what he was speaking of, but there were several miracles that came to mind. Brigie's inward calm and peace, her trusting acceptance of a new life opening up, the closeness of us all with each other and with her. These were blessings which would have seemed impossible under such circumstances. He could understand the desperate feeling, he said, that one wanted to *do* something to save the physical life: it was natural at this stage. I cannot remember what else he said, but the reassuring message was that the quiet way was right. It had been another very helpful talk. He blessed Brigie and was gone.

Mary Ann rang to say that she and Jenny were in the area and would like to come. The last message to her had given good news: she was distressed to hear that Brigie was not so well again, but they would come anyway. They arrived in the early evening and we left them to go in and see Brigie. Very soon we heard a movement: they were coming out, in tears. 'I can't bear to see her looking like that.'

We were still trying to comfort them when David, Martin and Kate came. All was very quiet and subdued and none of them stayed very long. Mark was in later, too.

By Wednesday the nursing had become very difficult again. Because we had a secure safe for the post office, diamorphine syringes were brought against the time when Brigie would perhaps be unable to take the 'cocktail', as Sister D. called it, orally. There was now the possibility of pressure points developing on her back. The nurse rubbed these with surgical spirit, but it was very hard to get Brigie into the right position now that she was so sleepy again. She suggested that Jane and I should get her into an upright position and support her there while she massaged. This is one time that Jane and I are ashamed to remember. Brigie was very weak, and we were tired. We managed to get her upright, but she had no strength at all, and very suddenly and shockingly, like a puppet deprived of its strings, she flopped—not right down because we were holding her, but the movement was both pathetic and ludicrous—and we laughed. As I think about it now, I am still shaken with the mixture of tears and laughter which assailed us then. It happened again and we were out of control once more. The operation was finally accomplished and we got her back on the settee. It was, no doubt, a release of tension for us, but what it did for Brigie I do not know. If she was aware of it, perhaps it was a sign that her two supporters were going on being themselves in spite of the strain, and perhaps there was something reassuring about that. And possibly it made her cross, remembering the furies long past, when she had fallen over and her siblings had laughed at her. If she knows about me writing this she might also remember her equal mirth when something discomforting happened to them. There were many times in the last two winters—good to think about now—when we were all sitting round the fire and memories were exchanged. And often when someone said, 'Remember that time when . . .' it was about such an event, with cross-accusations flying about.

Sister N. found the perfect solution for her back, a type of spray-on skin which protected her from rubbing and made the massaging unnecessary, so that this difficult manoeuvre did not happen again.

There was one other occasion that week when Jane and I were in gales of laughter, but Brigie was this time definitely oblivious. We had to support her on the bedpan. It was hard to get her on comfortably, and we were not very clever at it, especially as I had to lean over the settee back. The strain on our arms was considerable. It was important to us for it to be successful as it would save Brigie a good deal of discomfort later and give Jane a longer sleep—I had to wake her for help at these times. With considerable satisfaction we got her finally sitting and then, instead of concentrating on the task as we hoped she would, she went off into ecstasies about a waking dream that she was having. There she was sitting on the bedpan, saying in her most delighted voice, 'It was absolutely beautiful—absolutely beautiful! Come on—clap! clap! It was absolutely beautiful!' And she insisted on holding each of our half-free hands and clapping them together, while again we were in paroxysms of discomfort and mirth at the incongruity of it all. She could not tell us what was so beautiful, but it was a marvellous experience for her— and we were stiff for ages afterwards. Professional nurses would have been much more efficient, but I know, for all our shortcomings, Brigie was glad that it was us looking after her.

Some of her friends had been to see her while she was feeling better, but now we knew we had to tell them again that she was sinking. Once more, they must have the chance to say goodbye to her, and we braced ourselves for these distressing final visits, even though we still cherished the hope that she might rally again. I rang several mothers of Brigie's friends, and then Gladys and Dick, and arranged for them to come the following Wednesday, leaving it till then so that they could go to the short service of silent prayer which Ruth was leading every week now. Local people had asked for this service, and Jane and I wanted to go this Wednesday if Brigie could be left for a short time. Andrew would look after her, and we went down with Margaret Walker. We met in the choir-stalls and I was moved to see a number of friends. Ruth led a short meditation on the circle of prayer and the wider circle of those who were with us in spirit; on the space created inside that circle where love and power were concentrated. That time of quiet prayer together was very helpful. We got back to find that Andrew had managed to help Brigie on to the commode: they were both proud of this feat. Her inhibitions were going, and it was good that her brother could do this for her, a previously very private undertaking.

There was still some conversation with Brigie—moments of lucidity and communication for which we were very thankful. She was delighted one day at a blue-tit which came to the window, and Andrew hung some peanuts outside there so that she could see them more often. I went in to her one night when Jane and Michael were there: he was wearing the jeans which had been sprayed with acid and which showed a goodly expanse of leg.

'Brigie says she's going to mend my trousers tomorrow.' He sat and grinned at her. 'And mind you don't forget this one,' pointing to the largest hole of all. She smiled her enjoyment. Sewing seemed to be on her mind for several days, possibly going back to the time earlier when Jane had solved a problem of sewing a button back on to one of her nighties. These small matters seemed to take on threatening proportions for her when she was most confused, and she became very worried at this time about the ring Mark had given her. Was it an engagement ring? she asked me anxiously. I assured her it was not; it was simply a present from Mark, and she did not wear it on her engagement finger. Anyone would ask you first, I said, before they gave you an engagement ring.

On Thursday morning Margaret Walker came into the shop. She had been thinking more about Brigie. She had suggestions about special diets which she had read about and said that Ron, her husband, could get supplies for us from some of the shops they knew in Manchester. She mentioned various products that she had heard were very effective. It was hard to know what to say: I was very grateful for her intense concern, but it would not be possible to persuade Brigie to take anything. I explained that she was again having just sips of fluid. We had considered diets early on, but the thing had moved too swiftly for us. Anyway, she said, she would leave some Vitamin E tablets to use, or not, as we thought fit. I did not doubt her knowledge of the subject, as I knew she had read widely on it, but I knew it would be unkind and ineffective to ask Brigie to take remedies at this stage.

It was Sister D.'s turn to look after Brigie. She had been telling me for days that I should get out of the house, even for ten minutes in the garden. It was important to get a break, she said. This time she insisted. She would come back in the evening and then G. and I would have to depart. There was no point in demurring: she was formidable in this mood. How she fitted arrangements like this into a busy life of family and work, I do not know. Eileen had made a pie for the family, and we went to Skipton and had a drink and then a rather indifferent meal for which we had to wait a long time. It all seemed very unreal, but in retrospect it was refreshing to have had a change. Sister D. had been jolly and involved with everyone while we were out, helping Michael with his homework—there were the encyclopaedias about to prove it. Kate had been with Brigie when we left, but by the time Joanne and her mother came Brigie was very tired and sleepy. I was sorry about this as they had a long journey for a short visit, but it was impossible to plan for Brigie's times of awareness. Robyn had been in during the afternoon with flowers for her, but Brigie had been sitting up in the armchair then and never felt like seeing people unless she was on her settee.

Later that evening she became irritated with me again, so

I asked her who she wanted with her. 'Not you, and not Geoffrey,' she said.

'Jane?'

'Yes, Jane, or Andrew or Michael, but not you.' I was becoming used to my dismissals by now, and had to be grateful that the other three were able to give her what she needed. The following day, when she was awake and peaceful, I said, 'It's absolutely lovely having a daughter like you,' and I gave her a kiss. It was the last real communication I had with her and her eyes smiled. Dr. K. came and confirmed that she was 'very poorly' again. He said he thought the dexamethasone had produced the temporary improvement: he had thought it would relieve the pressure of fluid on her brain, and now felt that it had reduced the fluid on her lung and liver as well. So he had found a medical reason after all. G.M. and Marilyn arrived in the afternoon, and Abigail and Janet after school. David, Martin and Kate were here in the evening. Brigie seemed very remote.

So remote, in fact, that we felt she would not miss us if Jane and I went out for a while on Saturday. We would go and get our hair cut: we were both feeling very scruffy by now, and also, I think, we both needed to withdraw a bit. Marilyn remembers that I explained carefully to Brigie what we were doing, but she did not show any awareness. She asked for us while we were out, but when Marilyn said that we would be back soon she went to sleep again. She had to be woken again for medicine, and G.M. held her up while Andrew gave it. It was difficult to swallow. 'Bloody hell!' said Brigie.

Soon after we got back, Mark came and sat with Brigie. She was very poorly indeed, and Maurice sensed this when he arrived to give her a blessing. We were all there—G., G.M. and Marilyn, Andrew, Jane, Mark and I—I think not Michael. With shock I heard Maurice saying the Nunc Dimittis: 'Lord, now lettest thou thy servant depart in peace, according to thy word . . .' It was impossible to tell whether Brigie heard him or not. We were all very shaken. There was a quick, kind word to us all from Maurice and then he was gone. We realised that Mark had experienced a terrible shock. I thought I had told him plainly that Brigie was dying, but until that moment he had not really known it. He sat in the kitchen with a drink saying over and over again, 'I didn't realise.' There was nothing we could do for his pain.

Several people were to tell me later that at about this time they experienced a great release of tension about Brigie. Carol Rawson, like many others, had been thinking about her all the time, and it was always in terms of 'Poor Brigie'. As she was getting a meal ready this day, she felt a sudden lifting of her pity, and a conviction that all would be well for Brigie: she did not need to worry any more. Margaret Walker had something of the same feeling: a sudden realisation that she should let go and relax for Brigie, and Helen Dagett, reading in bed at night with her mother, said abruptly, 'Mummy, Brigie's going to be all right. I know she's going to be all right.' Margaret thought she meant that Brigie was going to recover, and worried for her daughter's inevitable disillusionment, but in fact she accepted the eventual out-come calmly.

Sunday was G.M.'s birthday, a very subdued affair, but his present was there, a *Wisden* ordered by Brigie some weeks before, after she had checked with Marilyn which ones he still needed for his collection. She herself was unaware, we think: Sister N. said she was semi-comatose. It was impossible to move her, but we had to wash her and change her regularly. Andrew helped with this as well as Jane, and I woke them alternately at night when this was needed. She was sleeping for very long periods and hardly woke enough for us to give her the diamorphine. That was becoming a real problem: it could take half an hour to rouse her sufficiently to take the medicine and then it was a great struggle for her to swallow it, and one was not quite sure how much she had got. It was especially difficult at night, when she seemed even more unconscious.

G.M. and Marilyn left on Sunday night to go back to

Broxbourne the next day. Andrew took G. to the train on Monday morning. It was a very quiet, tense morning. Sister N. gave her a very small wash, not wanting to disturb her. The day was dominated by the difficulty of giving Brigie the medicine. She went for long periods, sometimes six hours, before restlessness indicated she was ready. It took long cajolling and talking to rouse her enough, and I felt guilty at having to disturb her, but I knew that if she did not have it she would be in pain. She was obviously trying so hard, but the weariness was overpowering. Her eyes would open briefly, and seem to say, 'Please leave me alone,' and even when she opened her mouth a little the difficulty in swallowing was enormous. The syringes were ready, but she had always hated injections and we could not administer them anyway. The nurses, I felt, would not be able to come every time one was needed. It might mean going back to hospital and that would have been appalling for us all. I realise now that a way would probably have been found without moving her—we had been assured of every help in nursing her at home—but, at the time, it was a desperate anxiety. After one long struggle with the diamorphine on Monday I realised that Andrew, who had been sitting behind me while I knelt by Brigie, was very shaken and distressed.

'It was seeing her trying so hard to swallow,' he said through his tears.

I thought of Gladys, Dick and Lucy planning to come on Wednesday. I would suggest that as they had already said goodbye, and she might go at any time, they might decide not to come. There was no chance that she would know them. I explained all this to Gladys and she asked if it was better not to come 'just yet'. I had to say that it was not like that: she might die at any time. In that case, they said, they would come tomorrow (Tuesday). They would come by bus and get a taxi from Skipton. We arranged, though, that Andrew would meet them there.

Kate was sitting with Brigie when Maurice came on Monday evening. He said he had not expected to see her again. We were all there as he knelt beside her unconscious form and said a prayer which was unfamiliar to me:

Go forth upon thy journey from this world, O Christian soul,
In the name of God, the Father Almighty who created thee,
In the name of Jesus Christ who suffered for thee,
In communion with the blessed Saints, and aided by Angels and Archangels, and all the armies of the heavenly host.
May thy portion this day be in peace, and thy dwelling in the heavenly Jerusalem. Amen.

He was responding, he told me later, to an awareness of the 'heavenly company' and found this prayer most appropriate. I could fervently join him in asking that she might go, as I had done for the last two days. She was in a strange twilight area where there was just physical discomfort and no joy in remaining. We had to let her go. Now it was Kate for whom the full painful truth became clear. Like Mark, she had not absorbed the information until she heard the prayers, and she was terribly upset. She sat in the kitchen, and we tried to help her: when she was calmer she went home, declining company. She was brave, but I knew she was going to be very lonely without Brigie. Almost every night she had been here after work.

That night it was very difficult again to give Brigie the diamorphine. I was torn between the deep wish to leave her undisturbed, and to escape the emotional strain myself, and the necessity for getting her to take it. As a result, I made a misjudgment and left her too long. After I went to bed in the morning Jane had to wake me: Brigie was in distress. She was moving her head from side to side and moaning. Jane and Andrew had given her more diamorphine, but only one spoonful as it had been so difficult. I managed, at last, to get her to take some more, and we all sat, tense and miserable, hoping desperately that it would take effect quickly. It seemed hours, but was in fact about twenty minutes later when she gradually became quiet and still, and we knew she was out of pain. It had been very distressing, and I blamed myself: the only time at home when she had suffered bad pain, except in her leg when she went upstairs that night, and it was an indication of how bitterly painful it would have been without that strong drug.

Sister D. came in the early afternoon. She said she thought the time had come for injections. Brigie was too unconscious to take the drug orally and she assured us that Brigie would feel the needle very little.

'I'm just going to give you a little prick in your leg, my love,' she said. 'You'll hardly feel it.' That did seem to be the case. She made a slight movement and then was quite peaceful. I do not remember what Sister D. said about more injections, but in fact they were not needed.

Gladys, Dick and Lucy came about 3 p.m., very quietly, and went in to see Brigie one by one. I decided to get some pea soup from the freezer: it would be late when they got back to Ainsworth and the weather was very cool. This created muddle in our small kitchen and, as usual, took longer than expected, so I suggested that if they went on a later bus it would give them another hour, and they would also see Michael when he got back from school at 4.30 p.m. Dick's diary says: '. . . We did a short vigil each with Brigid: we were most upset and shocked to see how much she had deteriorated and how emaciated her features seemed to be . . .'

Jane was back with Brigie now, and I remember Dick was talking about the merits of pea soup and remarking that this was rather like it. 'But this *is* pea soup,' I said, and we had a laugh at a typically Grandad conversation: he, too, was being reassuringly himself. I went in to ask Jane if she would like some and Michael came home. I was getting Jane's ready when she came back and said,

'Mum, I think you'd better come.'

Nobody seemed to notice as I left the room. Brigie's head had moved to one side, facing us. She gave two slightly pronounced pants and then was very still. I thought she had died, but I could not be quite sure. I asked Jane to pass the mirror and held it to her: there did not seem to be any breath. We stayed there quietly for a few moments and Jane said, 'Her lips have gone very white.'

There was total stillness. It was over.

# 11

## Nunc dimittis

*I* felt fairly calm as I came back to tell the others and ask them
to come into the room. I wanted to say a prayer for Brigie:
just 'The peace of God which passes all understanding . . .'
and the blessing, the prayers which Maurice had said for her
so many times, and the same prayers which I had said for
Joan when she was near her death and for my father when he
died. I said the words now, but they were hardly audible
through the tears that suddenly overcame me. In the weeks
that followed it was often beautiful words that made me cry.
Dick's diary says: 'How pale and beautiful she looked in
death . . . we prayed together.' They stayed in the room but
there were things for me to do now, and that helped. I rang
Sister D. and the doctor, and brought the others back to the
kitchen. Dick spent a lot of time on his own, looking out of the
window. I thought it would be wrong for Andrew to drive at
this point, and Jane asked Stephen if he would take them
back to Skipton. I felt sorry for them having to make that
journey, but we did need to be on our own. I was glad they
had been here, though: Lucy reminded me that she had been
with us when Brigie was born, and it was good that she,
Brigie's godmother, had been there also when she died. I, for
one, was moving about like an automaton, numbed in feeling
but very shaky, I realised. I was glad that Jane drew my
attention to the marvellous sunset across the dale: there were

huge arcs of red cloud above the foss and the Brow, and it seemed to me like a welcome to Brigie. That lifeless figure still looked like Brigie but there was such a remoteness about her.

I badly needed to speak to G. and went up to the study: it was marvellous to hear him say that he would come at once. Andrew rang G.M. Gladys, Dick and Lucy left with Stephen and soon after Sister D. came: she had dropped everything and her presence gave us relief. I needed someone now to make decisions, even the small ones. She had already spoken to Raymond Harker, the undertaker, and she suggested a cup of tea (or was it a drink?) and she talked to us through our shock. I had forgotten how shocked and numbed one feels, even after long preparation for a death. I remembered now that even when Pompah died, a merciful release, I had cried and needed the cup of tea, the chat in the sister's office, and the kind and practical suggestions that followed. Now I was even more in need of some guiding energy. Sister D. organised the next step. We would wash Brigie and dress her ready for her burial. I had known all along that I wanted to do this, but I had not realised how shaky and feeble I would feel. Sister D. in fact did it all, but I helped. Jane ironed her special nightie, the lovely white embroidered one that Kate had given her and which she liked so much. I realised only when we washed her, and could move her freely now because it no longer hurt, just how pitifully thin she was. We made her ready and I brushed her hair, trying to give her fringe the flip-up which Brigie, when well, had always given it. The fringe was longer now, not touched since Val had given her its final cut, but I managed to make it look as if it had been on the old Brigie, swept-up and softening her forehead.

When we had done Sister D. helped me tidy the room (or rather I helped her) and she collected all the medicines and equipment no longer needed. At this stage Raymond came, and we sat in the room with Brigie and talked about her funeral. It was obvious he would fit in entirely with our wishes. He was much affected by the sight of her: he must have heard about her from James, his son. He would come the next day with her coffin, and she would stay here, in her own room, until she was buried.

While I was talking to him Sister D. was supporting 'the team' as she always called them, and I came back to find carrots and potatoes cooking for our meal. She had set Michael to putting the carrot tops in a dish of water to watch them grow more foliage. Dr. K. came while she was here: he spent time with her in the room while she was finishing the tidying. I thanked him before he left: 'You've been very good,' I said.

'I think you've been rather good, too,' was his response. Sister D. suggested that we all had a Mogadon that night and on the night of the funeral. She was very pressing in her offer to collect G. from the station, but Andrew was insistent that he would like to bring him home. She left, having done everything that was needed and much more besides, and we were stronger as a result. We all ate our meal in rather a daze. G.M. rang to say that they would drive up through the night, but I managed to persuade them to sleep and then come up in the morning. I rang Marion: she had heard, but she said afterwards how grateful she was for the call. They were thinking about us all the time and it was 'lovely to feel close to you' for just a few moments.

A message came from Ruth, a card with Michelangelo's painting of God creating Adam, the one hand strong and purposeful, reaching out across the abyss and almost touching the other. 'For Jan from Ruth,' it said, 'with my dearest love. Tues. Dec 1st 5.30 p.m. For Brigie now the tiny gap is closed between life and life. And when you reach out for her I think of her a bare finger-span away: except that, in another sense, while you live she is living as she was from the beginning, beneath your heart. For her there is no time till you are together.' She would be in church on Wednesday as planned.

Andrew and Michael left to collect G. I was sure Andrew was safe for driving and he very much wanted to go. It was a great help to have G. back. He went in to see Brigie. She still looked lovely with her hair curling over her shoulders, but so remote and still, and the room was very cheerless and bare without the fire and all the paraphernalia of the sick room.

We all needed to sleep. I suggested to Michael that he take his Mogadon.

'Not before I've got me boots off,' he said with a grin. We all laughed. He was quite deflated when he did take it. Instead of instant effect as he had expected, he felt quite normal: an anti-climax. We all had our Mogadons and drifted off to bed. For me, it was strange to think I would be staying there all night. We all, in fact, had a good night's sleep.

When I went in to see Brigie in the morning there was more of a change. She seemed even more distant and more like a waxen model of Brigie than Brigie herself. I had thought that I would feel very protective and attached emotionally to her body, but it was quite different. She seemed so completely *other*: it was not Brigie at all. She, herself, was away and this that was left was almost irrelevant. I still would not have had her body anywhere but at home, but I had no desire to sit with her, or be with her, because it was not *her*. Already I felt that she was with us, all about us, but not anything to do with that pale frame.

G.M. and Marilyn arrived in the late morning and spent some time in the sitting room. They were very shaken. Later Raymond came with the coffin, and Brigie went back to her own room again. She still looked peaceful, but more strange, surrounded by peach-coloured silk fittings. On the top of the coffin was a simple and finely-engraved plate:

Brigid Anne Moorhouse
December 1st 1981

Jane and I went down with Margaret to the church. There were several others there; the time was quiet and peaceful as we knelt in the choir-stalls. 'We meet,' said Ruth, 'in the silence of absence . . .' There were prayers for Brigie and for us, and we left. Words were not necessary: there was just a kind handshake and a kiss from them. I was very touched by their feeling. On the way back Margaret asked me if I would like them to postpone the Litton party planned for Saturday evening, the day of Brigie's funeral. I said certainly not: we wanted everything to go on as normally as possible. If any of us felt we could come, she said, even for a short time, it would be good.

Maurice came later in the day and we talked about the funeral. I had a clear, general idea: the emphasis should be thanksgiving—for her life, however short, and for her spirit, and for the closeness and love that we had all experienced. I was incapable of translating that into concrete suggestions, except that I wanted to sing the metrical Psalm 23, and 'Now thank we all our God' as G.M. had suggested and as G. had wanted at Joan's funeral. G.M. had other suggestions: Psalm 121, 'I will lift up mine eyes unto the hills . . .' and the hymn, 'Immortal, invisible, God only wise'. He had also brought Brigie's baptismal candle, which he hoped that her godfather Paul would light during the service. A day or two later he remembered Dylan Thomas's 'And death shall have no dominion', and Jane felt there was something in Eliot. G. knew the very passage—the last stanza of 'East Coker'. Gradually, after talks with Maurice and Paul and their talking to each other, it all came together. Paul would read the poems, and John Robinson, offering to cancel an engagement in Cambridge, would preach. Maurice had thought there would be too many clergy and offered to retire. We could not have that, and he agreed to link the service and take the graveside committal. In this way, we felt, all the distinctive spiritual contributions would be brought together.

G.M. had another suggestion. We had done everything for Brigie ourselves up to now. Could her two fathers and two brothers carry her in her coffin? I felt it would be very difficult for them to carry her on their shoulders, but Raymond said it would be possible—he would guide them—and he thought it was very good if the family carried out this service. G. would be glad to, but I wondered about Andrew and particularly Michael. They readily agreed though.

One practical problem was that they did not have anything to wear. Michael had gone to school on Wednesday as usual: it seemed best to keep to his routine. On Thursday they would go to Settle for jackets. Andrew rang from there to say they were about fifty pounds each. That was impossible, and we had to think again. The Oxfam or Shelter shop in Ilkley seemed a likely solution and on Friday Jane went with them. They returned successful—Andrew with a Hardy Amies tweed suit for six pounds fifty and Michael with one for five pounds. I thought Brigie would have a laugh if she knew about these economical arrangements.

G. thought out the details for which I had no concentration. He went to Skipton and registered Brigie's death. He said the registrar was almost in tears as she handed over the documents: it was one of the worst tasks she had had to do. He arranged for flowers and he and G.M. discussed the death notices. They spent a lot of time on the wording in order to include all this complicated family and the *Guardian* demurred at the unconventional form. G. had to ring up the paper and it was then accepted. He planned where we would all sit in church and talked to Tom Horner about the music. His quiet, methodical attention to detail gave me much reassurance. G. said late on Thursday afternoon that he would like to go down to the church and anyone who wanted to join him was welcome. He and I, G.M. and Marilyn went together: we went inside and they had a look round the building, and then we knelt down and were quiet together for a few minutes. After the time of constant phone calls and seeing people, it was good to be still and think of Brigie lying so still now, but so important to all of us, and to pray for her peace.

I was very touched to hear on Wednesday that John would come from Sweden for the funeral: that was a marvellous gesture of solidarity. Helen, with Tim, would come too, on Saturday morning, and old friends from Hertfordshire, Jenny and John, on Friday night. Eileen had offered hospitality overnight to any of our friends. G.M. would pick Paul up at Leeds at 10 a.m. and he would have to read the poems on the way as he did not know them. The anxiety was that the train would be late: the timing was tight for a noon service. There were to be tea and sandwiches at the Falcon afterwards and a meal here for those coming from a distance. The odd touches of humour helped me that week: as I was weeping over my cooking on Friday, Jane came through.

'Oh dear,' she said, 'you're crying into the lasagne. Don't put too much salt in it!' They were all very good at giving me a hug when I was overcome, and they reached for the tissue box yet again and thought how lucky we were to have a shop: otherwise there would surely have been many a tissue crisis.

John came on Friday afternoon: G. and Andrew fetched him from Ringway. It was good to have his big, strong hug. The same from Jenny and John: how reassuring and warming to see old friends. They brought messages and cakes and flowers from friends in Herts. The house was full again. G. did the post-office balance as he had done for weeks, and took all the documents to Arncliffe. We had been open as usual in the mornings, but people had been very considerate and came only if they had to. The post office would be closed on Saturday.

Helen and Tim came fairly early in the morning: they had set off from London at 4 a.m. We had some breakfast together, and then Jenny and John came to help, and Marilyn too. G.M. had gone to Leeds. We were all feeling very tense and it helped to have something to do. Concentration was still not easy, and I was glad of friendly people about to make suggestions. I very much hoped to be calm in public, and Jane did too, but we took a good supply of tissues just in case. Michael was fidgety and quiet, and Andrew nervous too about the carrying, but in another sense I was glad that they were to have this involvement and work to do. We went to get changed and the 'new' clothes gave us all a giggle. They looked very smart and it was hard to recognise Andrew in a suit. It was just as well that I had recently bought Michael a pair of black cords: his suit trousers were ludicrously big.

The wreaths had arrived during the morning: white and gold from G. and me, 'For our brave and spirited daughter with all our love'; gold lilies from G.M. and Marilyn, 'You are rare—and are missed'; and red, purple and white from Jane, Andrew and Michael, 'For our courageous sister who has taught us many things.'

We all assembled in the kitchen and Raymond arrived with the hearse. It was a dry day. He assured G. and Andrew and Michael that they would manage Brigie's coffin very well, and he would be there to help. His quiet confidence was very helpful. It was eleven thirty and we were waiting for G.M. and Paul. Marilyn was sure he would have rung if there had been a delay with the train. The minutes ticked by and we were getting very anxious. I wondered about taking something from the garden to put in Brigie's grave, but it seemed too sentimental. I wished afterwards that I had done so. If he was worried about the time, Raymond showed no sign: there was nothing we could do anyway, and as somebody said, 'They can't start without us.' I think we had a drink to steady our nerves. It was just after eleven fifty when G.M. and Paul got here: the train *had* been late as G. said it would be, and they must have had a fraught drive with Paul having to read the poems as well. He had the baptismal candle, and I took him into the sitting room for a quick change while the others brought the coffin down. I was very glad to see that he had his red cassock: Brigie would have liked that. (He had written to her, telling her about being appointed a Queen's Chaplain and how his congregation had given him this splendid robe which would have been too expensive for him.) I had not seen Paul for years: he looked very distinguished, the red surmounted with his now white hair. There was time for just a quick meeting with G. and then we had to go.

G., Jane, Andrew, Michael and I went first behind the hearse, then G.M., Marilyn and Paul, and Helen, Tim and John in their car. We felt more comfortable in our own cars than in the 'limousines' that Brigie had so relished at Pompah's funeral.

Jane looked back and saw Paul's robe hanging through the door; he had been in such a hurry to get in. She motioned to him through the back window, and then she had a laugh as he organised the rearrangement: 'He's put the candle in his mouth!'

Michael was very quiet, and we looked at Brigie's coffin ahead of us and thought of her making her last journey down the dale, this dale that she had loved so much and longed to live in. Now it had all passed away from her, and I knew that something even better was around her now. The hearse drew up to the church gate and we parked opposite. I could see Garnett and the other gravediggers waiting inside the old vicarage gates. Gladys and Dick and Lucy were in the porch, and they came down the path to join us. The bearers had a few minutes to adjust to their burden and we followed them slowly up the path, Jane and I, Gladys and Dick, Marilyn and Lucy, John, Helen and Tim. Maurice met us at the door: he had already spoken to the congregation and said that we wanted this to be a service of thanksgiving. I heard afterwards from Carol Rawson how relieved she had been to hear that: a conventional funeral service would have been so out of place.

I was very much aware of us as a family as we entered the church, those carrying their daughter and their sister, arms linked and strong around each other, and round her, and those of us walking behind. There was a great body of people, but I was conscious of just one or two familiar figures. Maurice was saying: 'I am the resurrection and the life, saith the Lord: he that believeth in me, though he were dead, yet shall he live and whosoever liveth and believeth in me shall never die.'

They rested Brigie's coffin at the bottom of the steps with the flowers brightly heaped upon it, and we took our places: Jane, Andrew, Michael, G. and I on the right, G.M., Marilyn, Gladys, Dick and Lucy on the left.

As we spoke the words of Psalm 121, 'I will lift up mine eyes unto the hills . . .' I thought of the limestone cliffs around us, and how Brigie had loved them. There was assurance here as well, 'The Lord shall preserve thee from all evil: yea, it is even He that shall keep thy soul'; reiterated in the strong and confident words of Psalm 23, sung to the tune Crimond. Here were the green pastures and the quiet waters that my grandfather was talking about, so I was told, as he lay dying. It was good to affirm in that beautiful sound the trust which Brigie herself had found, and I believed it was true for her to declare: 'And in God's house for evermore, my dwelling place shall be.' There were prayers led by Maurice, and then Paul came to the top of the steps and read 'And death shall have no dominion'.

And death shall have no dominion.
Dead men naked they shall be one
With the man in the wind and the west moon;
When their bones are picked clean and the clean
                              bones gone,
They shall have stars at elbow and foot;
Though they go mad they shall be sane,
Though they sink through the sea they shall
                              rise again;
Though lovers be lost love shall not;
And death shall have no dominion.

And death shall have no dominion.
Under the windings of the sea
They lying long shall not die windily;
Twisting on racks when sinews give way,
Strapped to a wheel, yet they shall not break;
Faith in their hands shall snap in two,
And the unicorn evils run them through;
Split all ends up they shan't crack;
And death shall have no dominion.

And death shall have no dominion.
No more may gulls cry at their ears
Or waves break loud on the seashores;

Where blew a flower may a flower no more
Lift its head to the blows of the rain;
Though they be mad and dead as nails,
Heads of the characters hammer through daisies;
Break in the sun till the sun breaks down,
And death shall have no dominion.

It was strong and stark and defiant, a fitting commentary, I
felt, on Brigie's realism, her acceptance of death and refusal
to be defeated. Such an attitude must be impossible for her
school friends, behind us, to comprehend, and I hoped that
some of their tension would be released in the singing of
'Immortal, invisible, God only wise', with its full bodied tune
and words that soared and praised. Paul was reading again
after that from Eliot's 'East Coker':

Home is where one starts from. As we grow older
The world becomes stranger, the pattern more
                                        complicated
Of dead and living. Not the intense moment
Isolated, with no before and after,
But a lifetime burning in every moment
And not the lifetime of one man only
But of old stones that cannot be deciphered.
There is a time for the evening under starlight,
A time for the evening under lamplight.
(The evening with the photograph album).
Love is most nearly itself
When here and now cease to matter.
Old men ought to be explorers
Here and there does not matter
We must be still and still moving
Into another intensity
For a further union, a deeper communion
Through the dark cold and the empty desolation,
The wave cry, the wind cry, the vast waters
Of the petrel and the porpoise. In my end is my beginning.

Both readings had been strong and compelling, powerful statements of hope and triumph, and I trusted that all Brigie's young friends were catching something of the forceful message. For my part, tears were unthought of, and many of us were caught up into something which went beyond grief or sorrow. 'In my end is my beginning' led us on to continuity through new life and, remembering the spiritual insights and glimpses which Brigie seemed to experience in her last weeks, I felt that we were expressing a reality for her.

The moment for lighting the candle had come. Maurice explained that Paul, her godfather, had given it to Brigie when she was baptised and he would place it now on her coffin. It shone and glowed among the flowers while John Robinson addressed us.*

His message caught the spirit of hope and deepened and enriched it. If there was one part above all others which people remembered afterwards it was 'If God is in the sunset, then He is in the cancer'; many were grateful for his directness and plain speaking, and he helped us to confront the evil and to see that it had been shot through and transformed into something strong and positive by love and prayer. The final hymn, 'Now thank we all our God', was a fitting communal expression of the sense of thanksgiving for all this grace. I, for one, sang it very fervently even though, at this point. I was close to tears.

The first part of the service was over: both Jane and I wished it not to end, it had been so strong and compelling. We moved out, and waited while the bearers rearranged themselves. G. told me afterwards that his arm had been numb and useless all this time after the awkward pressure of the weight, and they took the coffin in a different order at this point. Raymond had explained before that a coffin is carried with the weight, the head, at the back, and the feet in front. I had time to watch them now struggle and take the weight, their faces drawn and tight with concentration. It was a very

* Quoted in full in Appendix 2.

moving sight, all with their separate connections and love for Brigie working as a team, as we had been all along. We moved slowly down the nave behind them with the congregation singing the Nunc Dimittis: 'Lord, now lettest thou thy servant depart in peace, according to thy word . . .' Paul held the lighted candle cupped against the wind.

We stood around the open grave while they carefully and strongly lowered the coffin on its ropes with Raymond's unobtrusive help. I was so glad they were doing this last service for Brigie: it seemed to symbolise the fact that we had been with her to the end. As someone said afterwards, the family was actually laying her to rest. G. came back to me, and Maurice said the committal prayers.

I was suddenly conscious of the beautiful sound of the river behind us, and the rooks in the tall trees. What a quiet and peaceful place it was. G. gave me something to drop into the grave, and I wished then that I had brought something personal. Paul carefully dropped the still burning candle into the grave and Kate put in the posy that she had sent for Brigie and then walked quickly away. Mary Ann put something in. Most people were standing further off, moved and thoughtful, not wanting to intrude. I wanted to thank them all for being with us, but they began moving off. There was no time then to look closely at the mass of flowers lining the path and I must see people at the Falcon.

There were not as many there as I had expected, but many, like the girls as Miss Kent explained, had been too upset and needed to go home. I talked to Miss Kent, Mrs. Watkins and Mrs. Kilvington and several other teachers from the High School, Sarah and Bob and Kate, and Henry Heaton. He and Mary Miller had prepared the church for us: he had never seen the church so full, he said, and I wished I had been able to see more of those who had come. Miss Kent told G. that the school was going to establish a memorial fund for Brigie and every form would work for this next term. Elspeth had organised a very substantial table and her three-year-old Richard was helping with the sausage rolls. She told me that he had looked at Paul and asked her what Father Christmas was doing there. Paul was delighted and apologised for his lack of beard. David and Martin gave me a kiss before they left. Then out to more people in the hall, among them Colin and R.A.F. Dave; he told me how they had made a flying-suit for Brigie with her name on, in the hope that they would get her up in the helicopter. It had been a wonderful service, they said, very positive and strong. Val and Dennis were there, and Michael joined them. We left him there when we went: he needed a relief from the tension and it was time for us to go.

John and Ruth joined us and we were busy with drinks and lasagne. The room looked bright and cheerful again, not with the flowers of the sick room but with many beautiful and thoughtful gifts to us. Paul's time was limited. Stephen was taking him back to Leeds. He had time to go out into the garden for a few moments and see our surroundings. We stood there, looking up at the other side of the dale, at the foss and the Brow. It was unfamiliar country to him, and I hoped he would come back.

'Well, Jan, you've been very blessed in your family, I think.'

I thought of the four of them and knew he was right. As he got ready at the car he said, in a slightly surprised way, 'It's really been a joyful day, hasn't it?' And I realised with a slight shock that it was true.

G. suggested that we go back to the churchyard to see the flowers and collect the cards before it got dark. Kate, Jane and Andrew came too. The grave had been filled in and all the flowers heaped upon it. It was a beautiful sight, a mass of brilliant colour vivid against the grey of the church and walls and headstones. Many people had thought about Brigie, and especially touching were the posies from her friends: 'For my dear friend, Brigie, with my love, Rebecca', 'For a very dear friend', posy after posy, beautiful and delicate with tiny roses and dainty frills. 'Remembering the good times. John'. It seemed a pity to remove the cards, but rain, if it happened as it so often does up here, would have obliterated the words. Kate was composed and helpful and was able to identify many names for us.

Jenny and John left soon after we got back. It had been very good for me that they were here, and it was equally good for them, they said. The service had been 'inspiring'. In a way, they were the representatives of all the friends in Herts who had all been so concerned and caught up with us for weeks, and who felt very cut off and isolated. They would go back and tell the others that there had been a kind of triumph where there might have been disaster.

The Litton party happened that night. Jane, Andrew and Michael went, and I went later for a short time while G. was with John. Janet Beard told me later that it was so good to hear Andrew say, rubbing his shoulder, 'Cor, my arm doesn't half hurt with carrying that coffin!' How splendid, she thought, that he could talk naturally about it, and how good it had been, she said of the whole period, 'to see a family pulling together like that'.

On Monday, everything was very quiet again. Andrew took G. to the station and John to Manchester for his plane back to Sweden. Michael went to school. It was just Jane and I at home. At lunch time there was a letter from Mother Jane: I was tensely anxious to know about Sister Elvira, and went into the sitting room to read it by myself.

'My dear Jan,' it said. 'Thank you for telling us. Sister Elvira was there to welcome her as she went on November 22nd. She was aware to the end and able to take in what I told her you'd said about holding Brigie by the hand. Someone gave me this [card] when she died—and now it comes to you with all our love and prayers and alongsidedness, Jane.'

I wept with relief, and knew for sure then that my promise to Brigie that she would not be lonely would be fulfilled; with the soul of one of those loving women she would be safe. When I thought back on the dates, I realised that if Brigie had died when we first expected her to, it would have been before Elvira: that, to me, was one of the miracles that happened. It seemed to me then, and it still seems now, that one may not be granted what one feels to be one's deepest yearning, in this case Brigie's physical recovery, but one is given the strength and the circumstances to bear its denial.

We had all been through a very intense experience. We had seen the courage and spirit of Brigie, the bright and lively teenager who came to accept death with peace and trust, giving us love and strength all through. Physically worn and deeply grieved as we were, we came through it enriched and strengthened. The intense pain of parting is still with us, but there is, very importantly, what one of the sisters at Fairacres described: 'the strange blessing that seems to hide itself in all life's sorrows'.

# Postscript

In the weeks and months that followed there were these two distinct strands of feeling: the pain and grief that would suddenly overwhelm us and the high state of wonder as if we had been on a mountain top and had glimpsed a more profound reality that we had ever known before. The return to a kind of normality was painful, as Jane said, and for Andrew the effort of settling to work was hard 'because everything seems so superficial'.

I had time to look back on the early dread, and to consider what had made this outcome possible. The place had been very important: Brigie was at home for much of the time and especially for the last three and a half weeks. Not only that, she was in the sitting room, the focal place for the family. This was where she was happiest and knew she belonged. We could all be natural here and responsive when needed, and she was secure. Just as important, she was still part of the community. I often thought, seeing a large group sitting round her, or our customers who are also our friends popping in and out to see her (she was only a few steps away from the post office) that it was a very public dying. Her school friends could come too because their families were prepared to drive forty miles to give them perhaps just ten minutes with her. As one of them said to me, 'She must know she's loved with all these people coming.'

In several ways the house was inconvenient for the task. Downstairs we had just a very small kitchen (an extension was planned but had not happened then) and the modest sitting room. What would have been a dining room is, in fact, the small post office and shop. Often visitors had to duck beneath the damp washing hanging in the short passage, because it was the only place we had for drying on a wet day. None of this was important, compared with the immense priority of having Brigie at home.

We would not have managed without the backing of the medical and nursing professionals, themselves prepared to travel long distances each day, and to give us all the help we needed and more. There were enough of us too, 'the team' as Sister D. always called us, to ensure that no one became exhausted beyond endurance. We were profoundly grateful that Brigie had not been subjected to amputation and treatment. That would undoubtedly have caused terrible distress and would have deprived her of her last, very good summer, and it would have failed to save her life. As it was, she died a whole person, with her own self still intact.

Friends around us made a great contribution, those who brought logs for the fire and meals ready cooked, or did the ironing and the shopping, which eased the physical load and gave us more time to spend with Brigie. There was not just the practical support, important as that was: there were also those nearby who could talk to us so helpfully and give Brigie and us the support of their prayers and love, and so many others far distant in space but close in spirit. Their contribution was transmitted to others as well; many people spoke afterwards of the calm and faith they felt here which helped them to accept and trust. Brigie's peace was the real miracle, the looking forward to 'going home'.

Only in memory now the chirpy voice saying 'Hi, Mum!' as she came round the corner of the barn, but I believe that voice is transformed into the praising of her dream. 'Suffering and death for the young is a mystery . . . but He is love.' The mystery remains, but we learned much more about the love.

# Appendix 1

―――――◇―――――

## The Tillich Meditation

We all know that we cannot separate ourselves at any time from the world to which we belong. There is no ultimate privacy or final isolation. We are always held and comprehended by something that is greater than we are, that has a claim upon us, and that demands response from us. The most intimate motions within the depths of our souls are not completely our own. For they belong also to our friends, to mankind, to the universe, and to the Ground of all being, the aim of our life. Nothing can be hidden ultimately. It is always reflected in the mirror in which nothing can be concealed. Does anybody really believe that his most secret thoughts and desires are not manifest in the whole of being, or that the events within the darkness of his subconscious or in the isolation of his consciousness do not produce eternal repercussions? Does anybody really believe that he can escape from the responsibility of what he had done and thought in secret? Omniscience means that our mystery is manifest. Omnipresence means that our privacy is public. The centre of our whole being is involved in the centre of all being; and the centre of all being rests in the centre of our being. I do not believe that any serious man can deny that experience, no matter how he may express it. And if he had had the experience, he has also met something within him that makes him desire to escape the consequence of it. For man is not equal to his own experience; he attempts to forget it; and he knows that he *cannot* forget it.

# Appendix 2

*John Robinson's Address*

*I* feel very conscious of being the wrong person to give this address. Because I have been cut off in Cambridge for the past eight weeks I don't feel I really got to know Brigie when it mattered most. On the other hand, I have been conscious of living with it on the telephone every night and have felt very close.

What can one say? One's instinct is, like Job faced with such mysteries, to shut up, or, like the Psalmist, to keep silent even from good words.

But let me try to say two things, simple things but not easy things. The first is negative and the second positive.

The first is that God is not outside this any more than he is outside anything else. If God is in the sunset, then he is in the cancer. That may seem a terrible thing to say. But there are many faces of God, terrifying and benevolent. I couldn't possibly believe in a God who is above it all, watching it from the outside, let alone 'sending' it. That would make him a very Devil. As I see it, however dimly, the natural processes of the sub-human creation, some beautiful, some ghastly, some simply statistical and neutral, are not in themselves expressions of intention, God's or anyone else's. But they are part of the dark, mysterious, agonising and yet purposive forces of evolution leading up to man and to Christ and to the summing up of all things *as love*. That purpose of vanquishing vanity by love can only be wrought, as Christ wrought it, at the last through wood and nails. We cannot see meaning, let alone purpose, in the cancer, but we can, through Christ the prince of life, wrest meaning from it. The power of love as the source, ground and goal of all creation, which is what I mean by God, is not outside it but in it, taking it up into itself, and through suffering transforming into personal purpose what would otherwise be sheer purposeless futility.

Then secondly (very positively) not only is God in it but we too are called to share in that process, of creating—and receiving—love and goodness out of evil. Paradoxically, I believe that those who have been closest to Brigie, and that means, in spirit if not in flesh, most of us here, can testify to a great sense of thanksgiving. I believe that as a result of all we have been through our lives have been deepened, we have become closer and more open, not simply to each other (though that is a great grace that we would not have won by trying) but to the power of love by which all our lives are grounded and given meaning. We have touched the hem of 'the most real thing in the world' which, said St. Thomas Aquinas, is 'what all men call God'. And we have known that it is stronger than the grave, that it cannot be defeated or terminated by death or it would not be what we have known it to be.

Brigie has done that for us, or rather God has done that for us through Brigie. Her life has not been in vain, and in a short time she has brought grace to many; and her life is not snuffed out, even though what St. Paul calls the tent that houses us now decayed for her more quickly than for most. Indeed for her the powers of growth and the powers of diminishment met and contended together. That is why, at her age, the cancerous cells raced and multiplied as rapidly as the healthy. For most of us the one stage comes lingeringly, perhaps lovingly, after the other. But however it comes we all go out, not into nothing but into God. That is our sure faith and certain hope, which the pain and love of the last few weeks actually strengthen rather than weaken.

Let me end with a passage which expresses this to me most poignantly. It was written by an old man facing the running down of his powers after the exhilaration of youth and praying to find God in the processes of diminishment and death as much as in the exuberance of growth. I read from the French scientist and seer Teilhard de Chardin (*Le Milieu Divin*: pp. 69f.). It is a meditation we can all make our own whatever our age.

'It was a joy to me, O God, in the midst of the struggle, to feel that in developing myself I was increasing the hold that you have upon me; it was a joy to me, too, under the inward thrust of life or the favourable play of events, to abandon myself to your providence. Now that I have found the joy of utilising all forms of growth to make you, or to let you, grow in me, grant that I may willingly consent to this last phase of communion in the course of which I shall possess you by diminishing in you.

'After having perceived you as he who is "a greater myself", grant that when my hour comes, that I may recognise you under the species of each alien or hostile force that seems bent upon destroying or uprooting me. When the signs of age begin to mark my body (and still more when they touch my mind); when the ill that is to diminish me or carry me off strikes from without or is born within me; when the painful moment comes in which I suddenly awake to the fact that I am ill or growing old; and above all at that last moment when I feel I am losing hold of myself and am absolutely passive within the hands of the great unknown forces that have formed me; in all those dark moments, O God, grant that I may understand that it is you (provided only that my faith is strong enough) who are painfully parting the fibres of my being in order to penetrate to the very marrow of my substance and bear me away within yourself.' Amen.